Men, Masculini

Men, Masculinities and Health

Critical Perspectives

Edited by

Brendan Gough

and

Steve Robertson

palgrave
macmillan

First published 2010 by
PALGRAVE MACMILLAN

Palgrave Macmillan in the UK is an imprint of Macmillan Publishers Limited, registered in England, company number 785998, of Houndmills, Basingstoke, Hampshire RG21 6XS.

Palgrave Macmillan in the US is a division of St Martin's Press LLC, 175 Fifth Avenue, New York, NY 10010.

Palgrave Macmillan is the global academic imprint of the above companies and has companies and representatives throughout the world.

Palgrave® and Macmillan® are registered trademarks in the United States, the United Kingdom, Europe and other countries

ISBN-13: 978–0–230–20311–2   hardback
ISBN-13: 978–0–230–20312–9   paperback

This book is printed on paper suitable for recycling and made from fully managed and sustained forest sources. Logging, pulping and manufacturing processes are expected to conform to the environmental regulations of the country of origin.

A catalogue record for this book is available from the British Library.

10 9 8 7 6 5 4 3 2 1
19 18 17 16 15 14 13 12 11 10

Printed in China

BG: For Majella, Finn and Darcy

SR: For my big brother, Gaz

CONTENTS

Foreword

Over the last 20 years or so a considerable body of research has accumulated which focuses on the thorny issues surrounding men and their health. Much of this research developed from the powerful legacy of earlier feminist research which had highlighted the ways in which social structures and expectations (or more broadly the social relations of gender) 'made women sick' (Doyal 1995); a smaller body or research on men's health was framed as a backlash to earlier research on women's health as some claimed that men had been 'ignored' for too long. Whatever their motivations, from the 1980s onwards many people began to turn their attention towards considering men as gendered beings, influenced in no small part by key theorists such as who problematised the whole concept of 'masculinity' (e.g. Connell 1987; Hearn and Morgan, 1990; Connell 1995). Through the 1990s and beyond, a fascinating stream of empirical investigation increasingly focused on the intimate but sometimes elusive links between masculinity and health. This edited collection illustrates just how far this area of research has come.

Why should we care about men, masculinities and health? A starting point for many people is the fact that, in almost all countries of the globe, life expectancy for men is shorter than it is for women, despite the social and economic privileges that many men retain in many of these societies. This 'deficit' in life expectancy is often 'explained' by men's propensity to adopt more 'risky' and health-damaging behaviours or to delay seeking treatment for symptoms of ill-health (see, for example, Courtenay 2000), both commonly invoked as common ways through which men can demonstrate they are 'real' men. However, more recent research suggests that the adoption of over-simplistic, monotonic explanations of the link between men, masculinity and ill-health is unlikely to help improve the physical, mental and emotional health of boys and men (or indeed of girls and women, as they too of course are a part of and affected by the ways in which any society produces, reproduces, valorises or rejects various 'versions' or practices of masculinity). If we want to move forward in this field, a more critical approach is needed. That is why this book is so valuable and so well-timed.

The book is edited by two of the most well-respected scholars in the area of masculinities and health. Both here, and through their past research, Brendan Gough and Steve Robertson have been rigorous in bringing a more critical focus to the interrelationships between masculinities and health. In this stimulating collection they have not just concentrated on diseases of the male body. Whilst much has been learnt from earlier studies of men's experiences of such illnesses of prostate and testicular cancer, the breadth of the chapters in this collection has succeeded in raising wide-reaching issues about the conceptualisation, conduct, meaning and interpretation of research on men (or gender) and health. Many of the chapters draw on the authors' use of qualitative methods to research men's experiences of common causes of ill-health, mortality and distress, such as Broom's chapter on prostate cancer and Galdas' chapter on cardiac chest pain. It is excellent to see that this is accompanied by a thoughtful chapter discussing the ways in which the interview may encourage or discourage men from expressing their own understandings of health and their lives as men, and a critical view of some of the dilemmas about targeting health promotion material at men. There is a refreshing focus on less researched issues too, such as the increasing 'recognition' of depression in new fathers (which raises questions about the origin, meaning and prevalence of post-natal depression). The book also includes chapters examining pervasive images from the popular media and groups of men who are often overlooked (older men and men from ethnic minority groups). Throughout the key word is 'critical'; chapter by chapter the book draws attention to the complexities, ambiguities and apparent contradictions evident in men's discussions of their health (e.g. Robertson's 'Don't care/should care' view of men's health, which Lee portrays as 'Don't care/can't care for older men caring for dying wives). This makes the book a stimulating and thought-provoking read as well as a good resource for references on many aspects of empirical and theoretical writings on men and their health.

Because it draws all these strands together, this book will be valuable for anyone interested in research on men's health. It will also be invaluable to those interested more broadly in sociological or psychological studies of gender. Many of the chapters will also provide valuable food for thought for health professionals and policy makers or indeed anyone who is interested in how to move forward thinking about how we can harness some of our enhanced understandings of gender and health to begin to provide services or design interventions that incorporate these more nuanced understandings of the ways in which the social world influences the well-being of men.

Professor Kate Hunt
MRC Social and Public Health Sciences Unit
Glasgow University

Men, Masculinities and Social Theory (Ed J Hearn, D Morgan. Routledge, 1990)
Handbook of Studies of Men and Masculinity (Ed M Kimmel, J Hearn, RW Connell. Sage, 2004)

ACKNOWLEDGEMENTS

Thanks to those critical friends who have commented on draft papers on men's health and masculinities over the years, and who have indirectly contributed to this book, including Mark Conner, Murray Drummond, Sarah Grogan, Antonia Lyons, Anna Madill, Majella McFadden, Steve Robertson, Sarah Seymour-Smith, Alan White.

B.G.

Thanks to all my 'men's health' friends, colleagues and activists, too numerous to mention, who have kept me sharp and challenged over the last fifteen years. Thanks also to my 'blokey' mates, especially Andy, Dodge, Ed, Kitty and Les, who teach me so much about the contradictory nature of men's lives and always continue to surprise with their generosity of spirit.

S.R.

The authors and publishers would like to acknowledge the following:

The material in Chapter 1 is an amended version of an article first published by Elsevier Press: Lohan, M. (2007), 'How might we understand men's health better? Integrating explanations from critical studies on men's health and inequalities in health', *Social Science & Medicine*, 65(3), 493–504.

The writing of Chapter 4 was made possible by the generous career support provided by a Canadian Institutes of Health Research (Institute of Gender, Sex and Health) New Investigator award and a Michael Smith Foundation for Health Research Scholar award. The vignettes shared in the chapter are drawn from the author's doctoral research and projects funded by the Canadian Institutes of Health Research (Institute of Gender, Sex and Health) – *The role of prostate cancer support groups in health promotion*; *The role of South Asian men's groups in men's health behaviours* and *Families controlling and eliminating tobacco* (FACET). Special thanks are due to Melanie Phillips for her assistance, edits and thoughtful reviews of the earlier drafts of this chapter. Thanks also to Mary Kelly for her feedback in finalising the chapter.

The material in Chapter 5 is an amended version of an article first published by Sage Publications Ltd.: Seymour-Smith, S. (2008), '"Blokes don't like that sort of thing"', *Journal of Health Psychology* 13(6): 785–97.

Chapter 6 emerged from the ESRC Growing Older Programme: Older Men: Their Social Worlds and Healthy Lifestyles L480254033. The authors of the chapter would like to acknowledge the invaluable comments and guidance of Professor Sara Arber, who was the award holder of the above research project.

The material in Chapter 8 is an amended version of an article first published by Elsevier Press: Williams, R.A. (2007), 'Masculinities, fathering and health: the experiences of African-Caribbean and white working class fathers', *Social Science and Medicine* 64(2); 338–49.

The author of Chapter 9 would like to acknowledge Frank Furedi and Dana Rosenfeld for their thoughts and comments on earlier drafts of the chapter.

The material in Chapter 10 is an amended version of an article first published by the Men's Studies Press: Broom, A. (2004), 'Prostate cancer and masculinity in Australian society: A case of stolen identity?', *International Journal of Men's Health* 3(2): 73–91.

Every effort has been made to trace all the copyright holders, but if any have been inadvertently overlooked the publishers will be pleased to make the necessary arrangements at the first opportunity.

NOTES ON CONTRIBUTORS

Alex Broom is a Senior Lecturer in the Faculty of Health Sciences, University of Sydney, Australia. He has researched health issues in New Zealand, Australia, the UK, India, Pakistan and Sri Lanka. He is currently Deputy Director of the Australian Research Council Key Centre for Asia Pacific Social Transformation Studies (CAPSTRANS). His recent books include: *Men's Health: Body, Identity and Social Context* (Wiley-Blackwell, 2009), *Therapeutic Pluralism: Exploring the Experiences of Cancer Patients and Professionals* (2008) and *Traditional, Complementary and Alternative Medicine and Cancer Care* (2007).

David Buchbinder holds a Personal Chair in Masculinities Studies at Curtin University of Technology in Perth, Western Australia. He has edited *Essays in Masculinities Studies 2002*, a collection of undergraduate essays on masculinity; he has published two books, *Masculinities and Identities* (1994) and *Performance Anxieties: Re-presenting Men* (1998); and he has published widely in the area of masculinities studies, focusing on the cultural representations, across various genres and media, of men, masculinities and male sexualities. He has begun work on a third book on masculinity, provisionally titled *Malestrom: Masculinity at the Abyss?*

Kate Davidson is a Senior Lecturer in Social Policy and a co-director of the Centre for Research on Ageing (CRAG) at the University of Surrey, UK. Kate has a background in nursing and her particular areas of expertise are qualitative research with older people, focusing on their health and social relationships, especially of older men. She has published nationally and internationally and is co-editor with Sara Arber and Jay Ginn of *Gender and Ageing: Changing Roles and Relationships* (2003) and with Graham Fennel of *Intimacy in Later Life* (2004). She was President of the British Society of Gerontology from 2008 to 2010, and a Trustee of the Centre for Policy on Ageing.

Murray Drummond is an Associate Professor in Physical Education Studies at Flinders University, Adelaide, Australia and an Adjunct Associate Professor (men's health) in the School of Medicine at the University of Adelaide. He has a special interest in men's health and men's body image in particular and co-ordinates the only tertiary course in Australia that is solely dedicated to men's health. He has been the Chief Investigator of numerous qualitative men's health research projects spanning issues relating to male body image, prostate cancer and gay men's health. He sits on the editorial board of the *International Journal of Men's Health, Men and Masculinities, THYMOS: Journal of Boyhood Studies* and the *Gay & Lesbian Issues in Psychology Review*.

Paul Galdas is currently an Assistant Professor at School of Nursing at the University of British Columbia, Canada. He is a registered nurse in both the UK and Canada, with expertise in the area of medical cardiology. His research and scholarly activity have developed in the substantive area of help-seeking behaviour and men's heart health, with a theoretical focus on the social construction of masculinities among South Asian men.

Brendan Gough is Professor of Applied Social Psychology at Nottingham Trent University, UK. He is a critical social psychologist and qualitative researcher interested in gender issues, especially concerning men and masculinities. He has published various articles on gender identities and relations which draw upon discursive and psychoanalytic concepts, including areas such as sexism, homophobia and intersex. He has also published articles on ESRC-funded health-related research, such as alcohol consumption, smoking and aspects of men's health. He is co-editor of *Qualitative Research & Psychology* (Taylor & Francis) and *Social Psychology & Personality Compass* (Critical Psychology Section) (Blackwell).

Ellie Lee is Senior Lecturer in Social Policy at the University of Kent, UK. She researches, publishes and teaches in the areas of the sociology of reproduction, of health, and of the family. Her longest-standing research area is abortion policy and service provision. Her books include *Abortion Law and Politics Today* (Macmillan, 1998) and *Abortion, Motherhood and Mental Health* (Aldine Transaction, 2003), and more recently she has worked on influential studies about the provision of 'late' abortion and early medical abortion. Since 2004 she has also developed research projects about motherhood (specifically feeding babies) and parenthood (the contemporary medicalisation of motherhood and fatherhood). With Frank Furedi, she set up Parenting Culture Studies at Kent University in 2007 (www.parentingculturestidies.org) and in her spare time she co-ordinates www.prochoiceforum.org

Maria Lohan is a Lecturer in Health Sciences in the Nursing and Midwifery Research Unit of the School of Nursing and Midwifery at Queen's University Belfast, Northern Ireland. She is best known for her recent *Social Science and Medicine* article, 'How might we understand men's health better?' Her recent and current research centres on men's sexual and reproductive health, especially in understanding the role of men as clients and partners of clients in reproductive and sexual health services, e.g. men who have sex with men and partner notification, adolescent men and pregnancy decision-making and HIV and pregnancy decision-making. She is also co-author of *Social Theory, Health and Healthcare* (Palgrave Macmillan, 2009).

Robert Meadows is Lecturer in Sociology at the University of Surrey. For the last nine years his research has predominantly focused on issues surrounding 'sleep'. This research agenda has brought together interests in methods, sociological theory, the body, 'impairment' and (older) men's health. He has published in journals such as *The Sociological Review*, *Sociology of Health and Illness* and *Body & Society*.

John Oliffe is Associate Professor at the University of British Columbia, Canada. He worked as an emergency room clinical nurse specialist and taught undergraduate nursing programmes at Latrobe and Deakin universities while completing an M.Ed. His PhD and postdoctoral studies focused on men's psychosocial oncology issues. He holds Canadian Institutes of Health Research new investigator and Michael Smith Foundation for Health Research scholar awards. His men's health research programme includes nationally funded studies addressing prostate cancer, depression, South Asian immigrant men, smoking patterns of fathers and youth sexual health. He has also published articles exploring the use of masculinities and qualitative methods in men's health research.

Steve Robertson is currently Reader in Men's Health at the Centre for Men's Health, Leeds Metropolitan University, UK. He worked as a nurse and health visitor for over fifteen years before commencing a research career, completing his PhD at the Institute for Health Research, University of Lancaster. He has been publishing in the field of men's health, particularly in men's health promotion, for over fourteen years, and is author of *Understanding Men and Health: Masculinities, Identity and Well-Being* (Open University Press, 2007). He is best known for his work linking theories of masculinities to concepts of health and illness and has collaborated on published work in this area with colleagues in Australia, Canada and the USA.

Sarah Seymour-Smith is a Lecturer at Nottingham Trent University, UK. She is primarily a discursive psychologist but also draws upon conversation analysis, membership categorisation analysis and narrative analysis. Her research interests include masculinity and health, non-custodial fatherhood (especially groups such as Fathers 4 Justice), male sex offenders and long-distance learning.

Robert Williams is currently a Lecturer at the University of Birmingham, UK. He worked in health and social care for over twenty years, as a care assistant, nurse, district nurse, social worker, health visitor and health promotion officer. He won a Queen's Nursing Institute National Innovation Award in 1997 for research and development in men's health. His academic background is in sociology and social science, and he teaches sociology, public health and health promotion. His research interests are in the relationships between masculinities and men's health beliefs and practices, with specific interest in the links between masculinities, fatherhood and health.

INTRODUCTION: WHAT IS THE POINT OF THIS BOOK?

This is a fair question, especially given the ever-increasing media, policy and research attention devoted to men's health issues over the past twenty years or so. Of course, this attention to men's health is long overdue, considering enduring sex differences in mortality and the overrepresentation of men in statistics concerning major killers such as heart disease and cancers (see Box 1). While these trends can be partly explained through recourse to social class indicators (e.g. income, postcode, education), and biological factors can also be implicated (e.g. genetic predisposition), the role of gender remains significant. In other words, problems in men's health can and have been widely attributed to 'masculinity'. This thesis that masculinity is bad for men's health can be traced to Harrison's (1978) influential paper, 'Warning, the male sex role may be dangerous to your health', and it is a thesis which remains popular today, with, for example, dedicated media campaigns urging men to look after their health (see Gough, 2006). However, this pathologisation of masculinity masks the complex and sometimes contradictory nature of masculinity – or masculinities – which has been demonstrated in the wider literature on men and masculinity studies (e.g. Connell, 1995; Connell & Messerschmidt, 2005). It is only very recently that some researchers working in the field of men's health have taken on board this literature to produce more critical analyses of men's identities and lifestyle practices in relation to health contexts (see Robertson, 2007) – and we have invited a number of those people to contribute to this book. This book, then, is designed to showcase a range of contemporary theoretical and empirical contributions, emanating from a range of disciplinary (and interdisciplinary) settings and geographical locations (the UK, Canada, Australia) which foreground issues

Box 1 Men, mortality and morbidity: some headline figures

- Average life expectancy for men in the UK is approximately four years less that it is for women (Office for National Statistics, 2006).
- There are significant inequalities in life expectancy between men in terms of social class and geographical location (White *et al.*, 2005).
- Men's deaths exceed women's across a number of serious diseases; for example, men are twice as likely than women to develop and die from the ten most common cancers affecting both sexes (Men's Health Forum, 2004).
- Men in the UK are significantly more likely to be overweight and obese then women (Office for National Statistics, 2003).
- Men in the UK are less likely than women to consume the recommended five daily portions of fruit and vegetables, and are more likely to have a higher than recommended salt intake (Office for National Statistics, 2006).
- Men in the UK are more likely than women to drink above recommended amounts, to binge drink, and to take illicit drugs (Office for National Statistics, 2006).

of masculinities in diverse health-relevant arenas. Thus we have chapters from sociologists, social psychologists and media and cultural studies scholars as well as from former health professionals who have subsequently pursued research careers. As such, this book is aimed at a number of constituencies, including social and health scientists researching topics to do with gender, health and inequalities, health professionals involved in designing and enacting health promotion interventions with male client groups, and students and lecturers participating in courses where gender and/or health feature as key themes.

In explicating the various nuances and tensions pertaining to men's negotiation of health phenomena, qualitative research methods have been privileged by our contributors – in common with the wider men and masculinities literature. Of course, survey and experimental studies can be valuable in providing general information (e.g. sex-difference statistics on health service use) but the great strength of qualitative work lies in its capacity to illuminate lay understandings and practices within specified social contexts and therefore to complement and/or challenge quantitative data. Not surprisingly, interview methods are particularly in evidence in this book – as they are across qualitative research in health and social sciences – and yield fascinating, grounded and rich insights into men's constructions of health issues. Mass media representations of men and health, and health promotion generally, are attracting more research attention, and some authors focus on select media resources to underline points about contemporary masculinities within health contexts (Buchbinder in Chapter 2, Gough in Chapter 7, Lee in Chapter 9). A range of analytic methods, including thematic analysis, grounded theory and discourse analysis are deployed across the chapters, and Oliffe (Chapter 4) explicitly addresses key issues facing qualitative researchers working in the field of men's health. We think this variety makes for a stimulating and engaging text.

Rather than offer a consistent textbook perspective, then, our book is designed to showcase diverse theoretical and empirical contributions concerning the complex relationship between men, masculinities and health. We do not, for example, offer a once-and-for-all definition of 'masculinity'. Instead, we recognise that the term 'hegemonic masculinity' has been used in a range of ways – an issue which has attracted some criticism of the concept (see Connell & Messerschmidt, 2005). As editors, we were therefore left with two options relating to the use of the term: (1) to agree a definition ourselves in advance and have contributors utilise this definition within their chapters, or (2) to allow contributors to utilise the term as they will. In order to promote academic freedom, and not to stifle critiques that may rely on particular definitions of 'hegemonic masculinity', we have adopted the latter option. The term is therefore used and defined in slightly differing ways throughout. For example, it is identified as 'configurations of practice' by Lohan (Chapter 1) and Galdas (Chapter 12), as 'gender ideals' by Gough (Chapter 7) and implicated as 'sets of characteristics' by Lee (Chapter 9).

We have structured the book into three main sections. Part 1 deals with conceptual issues in the arena of men's health and begins with a perspective from media and cultural studies. In Chapter 1 Maria Lohan helpfully overviews two academic traditions which have variously informed men's health: critical studies on men and the inequalities in health literature. While both traditions have developed largely in parallel, Lohan makes a persuasive case for blending aspects of both in order to forge a more critical and sophisticated perspective on men's health issues. Then, in Chapter 2, David Buchbinder sets the scene for the book by drawing on the superhero genre in film to highlight both men's investment in invulnerability myths and their recognition of a more 'ordinary' status, and the extent to which individual men resolve these dual tendencies will, of course, imply health consequences. Our third chapter by Steve Robertson and Robert Williams adopts a more sociological tone through drawing on, for example, Foucauldian concepts (e.g. self-surveillance), notions of 'moral' citizenship (e.g. Lupton, Crawford) and embodiment (e.g. Williams, Turner) in order to speak to men's health. In this chapter accounts from men derived from the authors' and others' empirical studies are nicely counterposed with theoretical points in order to highlight some conceptual shortcomings and to argue for a critical, structuralist and embodied understanding of men, masculinity and health. Chapter 4 by John Oliffe then provides a reflexive piece which critically examines methodological (and other) issues in preparing for and conducting men's health research projects. This inventive personal reflection is neatly interspersed with vivid examples and illustrates some important challenges and opportunities in, for example, negotiating access to male patients and then striving to render the research encounter meaningful for both interviewer and interviewee.

In Part 2 the focus is on mundane accounts of health and well-being emerging from diverse locations – cancer support groups, older men, a health promotion publication and fathers from different ethnic backgrounds. Chapter 5, by Sarah Seymour-Smith, uses data from interviewees talking about their involvement in a testicular cancer self-help group to illustrate how men negotiate the delicate business of seeking (and offering) help. Her discursive analysis shows how gender is made relevant in various ways by her participants, not least in their efforts to construct their participation in self-help groups as 'legitimate'. The next chapter (6), by Kate Davidson and Robert Meadows, also focuses on another potentially threatening context for men: being 'older'. Through sampling a range of older men with respect to age, marital status and living arrangements, they highlight continuities in adherence to masculinised discourses over time while also drawing attention to important differences in self-care and lifestyles between men in different situations, with the role (or absence) of partners and extended families underlined as significant influences on older men's health. Chapter 7 by Brendan Gough turns to a men's health promotion text (on reducing obesity in men) in order to examine the construction and function of masculinities therein. His analysis suggests a reliance on stereotypical notions of masculinity (e.g. rational, autonomous actor) which, he argues, undermines the health promotion agenda since it is those very forms of masculinity which are implicated in men's poor health in the first place. The last chapter (8) in this section is by Robert Williams and focuses on a men's health project involving interviews with working-class fathers from different ethnic backgrounds. The accounts of these men are indeed varied but issues of material hardship and social prejudice (particularly racism) clearly impinge upon masculine identities and lifestyle practices, while at times other priorities such as pleasurable consumption and caring for children take precedence over health concerns.

Our third and final section comprises contributions which focus on how men are positioned – and position themselves – within illness contexts. While two chapters focus on classic 'male' diseases (coronary heart disease, testicular cancer), the other two deal with problems traditionally associated with women (post-natal depression [PND], eating disorders). Chapter 9 by Ellie Lee considers recent media and popular cultural attention directed at fathers and the 'hidden' issue of men struggling with undiagnosed PND. The medicalisation of men's vulnerability in relation to fatherhood is astutely discussed by Lee, with some question marks raised about the merits of such intervention and labelling; certainly, more research into men's experiences of parenting issues and encounters with health professionals is required here. Chapter 10 by Alex Broom addresses another point of male vulnerability: men diagnosed with prostate cancer. Based on interviews with male patients undergoing a variety of treatments, Broom highlights the central role of masculinities in shaping men's accounts and practices, most vividly illustrated by cases where urinary problems were not reported by men for 20 or more years due to lack of awareness and difficulties admitting to problems, and also the shared sense of humiliation reported by the (heterosexual) men concerning transrectal treatment procedures, implicitly linked to homosexual practice. The next chapter (11) by Murray Drummond also deals with embodiment issues, this time concerning men classified as suffering from body-image problems and/or eating disorders within sport and exercise contexts. Based on interviews with a range of men Drummond shows how, for example, sexual orientation and age mediate the accounts men provide when dealing with issues such as muscularity and fat consciousness, while also identifying the centrality of mass media images of the male body – and their reception – on some men's embodied identities. Our final chapter (12) by Paul Galdas considers interview data with men from South Asian and white British backgrounds who have suffered heart problems – ethnicity being a factor much overlooked to date in studies of men's health. In comparing accounts from both groups, Galdas is able to pinpoint differences in emphasis and gender-identity concerns, with recognising and divulging experiences of pain, early help-seeking within extended families, and respect for medical authority as normative practices for most South Asian men – themes not prevalent in the accounts of white British interviewees.

In sum, we feel we have put together a diverse and important collection which challenges some commonly held presumptions concerning masculinities and men's health practices and which makes a strong contribution to the field. While each chapter can be picked up as a stand-alone piece, it is clear that all authors are united by a commitment to critical work which draws upon men's accounts while paying attention to the local and wider social, material and cultural contexts in which men live and move.

REFERENCES

Connell, R.W. (1995) *Masculinities*. Cambridge: Polity.

Connell, R.W. & Messerschmidt, J.W. (2005) Hegemonic masculinity: rethinking the concept. *Gender & Society*, 19(6): 829–59.

Gough, B. (2006) 'Try to be healthy, but don't forgo your masculinity': deconstructing men's health discourse in the media. *Social Science & Medicine*, 63: 2476–88.

Harrison, J. (1978) Warning: the male sex role may be damaging to your health. *Journal of Social Issues*, 34: 65–86.

Men's Health Forum (2004) *Getting It Sorted: A Policy Programme for Men's Health*. London: Men's Health Forum.

Office for National Statistics (2003) *Social Trends 33*. London: Stationery Office.

Office for National Statistics (2006) *Social Trends 36*. Basingstoke: Palgrave Macmillan.

Robertson, S. (2007) *Understanding Men and Health: Masculinities, Identity and Well-being*. Open University Press: Buckingham.

White, C., Wiggins, R., Blane, D., Whitworth, A. & Glickman, M. (2005) Person, place or time? The effect of individual circumstances, area and changes over time on mortality in men, 1995–2001. *Health Statistics Quarterly*, 28: 18–27.

Part I

CURRENT ISSUES AND DEBATES IN THE FIELD OF MEN'S HEALTH AND MASCULINITY

1 DEVELOPING A CRITICAL MEN'S HEALTH DEBATE IN ACADEMIC SCHOLARSHIP

Maria Lohan

INTRODUCTION

For researchers interested in understanding men's health, and especially the recently reported phenomenon of men's poorer life expectancy relative to women's (White and Cash, 2004; Tsuchiya and Williams, 2005), there are two obvious literatures to mine. One is the rapidly developing studies of men's health arising from the study of men and masculinities. The second is the traditional study of inequalities in health. However, to date, there has been a schism between these two scholarships, and thus each is individually poor in their ability to provide an adequate explanatory framework for understanding the complexities involved in men's health research and practice. In this chapter, my intention is to develop an integrative explanatory framework of men's health from both men's health and inequalities in health literatures. The chapter is structured as follows. First, I situate studies of men's health in relation to the broader study of men and masculinities. Here I will argue that in order to create a link with inequalities in health research, men's health literature should be more firmly grounded in *critical studies on men* (CSM). Second, I briefly describe explanations current within the field of inequalities in health and I will suggest ways in which explanations from both scholarships (CSM and inequalities in health) can be integrated in order to develop a more critical approach to men's health.

MEN, MASCULINITIES AND HEALTH

In order to gain an overview of the men and masculinities scholarship, it can be instructive to distinguish between what Hearn (2004) calls *men's studies* and *critical studies on men* (CSM). While both men's studies and CSM developed in response to the broad-based women's movement, men's studies is based on an intellectual and community-based movement which seeks to reaffirm essentialist notions of manhood in light of the changing positioning of women in society. Men's studies writing (for example, Bly, 1990; Faludi, 1999; Phillips, 1999; Farrell, 1993) speaks of a 'men's crisis' or 'the crisis in masculinity' because, it is claimed, the natural order in gender relations has been severely threatened by women's 'misguided' attempts to transform the gender balance, resulting in men being increasingly disadvantaged in employment, education and intimate relations relative to women. The studies are often theoretically underdeveloped, relying on simplistic versions of Jungian and Freudian theories of 'true' male self-identity trapped behind layers of socialisation (Whitehead, 2002: 55). In essence, and at the risk of oversimplification, men's studies seek to celebrate male bonding and tell men they are OK, with no interest in promoting feminist theory or practice (Hearn, 2004).

CSM, by contrast, is the study of the gendered nature of men's lives which emerges primarily from within feminism and also gay and queer studies (see Hearn & Morgan, 1990 and Kimmel *et al.*, 2005 for an overview). The three key central markers of CSM are: (1) seeing gender as socially constructed; (2) challenging hegemonic masculinity; and (3) challenging gender power relations. Seeing gender as socially constructed, according to Kegan Gardiner (2005: 35), is the most significant achievement of twentieth-century feminist theory. It suggests that 'masculinity and femininity are loosely defined, historically variable, and interrelated social ascriptions to persons with certain kinds of bodies – not the natural, necessary, or ideal characteristics of people with similar genitals' (Kegan Gardiner, 2005: 35).

The concept of hegemonic masculinity (Carrigan *et al.*, 1985; Connell, 1995) has become central to studies of masculinities to capture the cultural dominance of particular ideals of masculinity, or configurations of gender practice, which operate in a particular context. Hegemonic masculinity represents the most exalted or leading version of masculinity which becomes embedded in institutional and cultural practices (for example, in politics, religion, urban space and popular culture) and acts to stabilise a structure of dominance in the gender order as a whole, such that alternate ideals of masculinity appear less legitimate (Coleman & Lohan, forthcoming). Nonetheless, it is theorised as a form of authority which is not essentialist or especially obdurate, but rather can be shaped by local conditions and resistances and is stabilised and destabilised by other types of power relations, such as social class and ethnicity (Connell, 1995; Connell & Messerschmidt, 2005). It is also a form of authority that ordinary men are not necessarily expected to reach up to but would, nonetheless, recognise as an ideal. Thus, the concept of hegemonic masculinity is also used to theorise hierarchies of power *between* men, and other types of masculinities, notably *complicit, subordinated* and *marginalised* masculinities (Connell, 1995). Turning now to challenging gender power relations, this is what Hearn (2004) describes as not just an interest in hegemonic masculinities but rather in the 'hegemony of men'. By this he means men's position of power in relation to women in society. CSM acknowledges that while power within and between gender relations may be complex, fluid and contradictory, it is imperative not to ignore the asymmetrical relationship between men and women and between masculinities and femininities in Western societies. It is to theorise men's lives in a way which does not re-exclude women and femininities (Hearn, 2004).

How do studies of men's health fit into the scholarship of men and masculinities? Academic studies of men's health do draw on the above CSM principles but do not always incorporate all three. I will re-examine men's health studies by drawing on these three principles forthwith. Studies of men's health have become a key site in which to study the social construction of gender in men's lives, reflecting on what it means to be a man in the modern world and how this might influence health practices. Reflecting the broader field of CSM, there has also been a move within studies of men's health from theorising masculinity in the singular to masculinities. This gives recognition to the multiple ways men live out masculine gender identities, as well as a growing recognition of intersecting aspects of masculine identities (such as sexuality, disability, ethnicity and social class) (Robertson & Williamson, 2005). Furthermore, studies of men's health have reflected the broader turn in feminist theory away from theorising gender processes in terms of passive socialisation into sex roles and towards theorising gender in terms of being an 'active' and on-going process (see Kimmel, 1987 for a critique of sex roles). In studies of men's health, men are actively seen to 'do' gender in the ways that men 'do' health (Saltonstall, 1993; Courtenay, 2000; Connell, 2000).

The concept of hegemonic masculinity has been highly prevalent in studies of men's health. Research on men's health has consistently drawn a link between a pattern of men's poor health behaviours, adoption of high health-risk activities and a reluctance to seek general health and medical advice with hegemonic cultural constructs of masculinities, defined in terms of male stoicism and masculine invincibility (for example, Moynihan, 1998; White and Johnson, 2000; White, 2001; Courtenay, 2000; Robertson, 2003; O'Brien *et al.*, 2005). However, while the concept of hegemonic masculinity is omnipresent in studies of men's health, the CSM focus on the need to *challenge* hegemonic masculinity is often missing (but see Gough 2006 for an exception). Much of the academic health professional research seeks a response to men's poorer health behaviours through changing the structures of the health services and especially in making health services more available and accessible to men. It is often assumed that contact with the health services and health education will consequently lead to behavioural/lifestyle changes. Thus, although the vast majority of men's health studies acknowledge the importance of forms of hegemonic masculinity as a key explanatory factor of men's poorer health and health behaviours, the focus is frequently on changing men's attitudes to health and health behaviours rather than *challenging hegemonic masculinity per se*. The categories of 'men' and 'hegemonic masculinity' have tended to acquire static and stable meanings in this type of research and health promotion (see Robertson & Williamson, 2005 for a review). CSM's health go further, seeking instead to challenge hegemonic gender relations in order to disrupt gendered health ideologies and practices (see: Sabo & Gordon, 1995; Connell *et al.*, 1999; Sabo, 1999; Segal, 1990; Doyal, 2000; Robertson, 2003).

Considerably less pervasive as an underlying theoretical principle in studies of men's health is an awareness of the relational power context of gender relations. Most distinctly, as Hearn (2004: 99) states, the 'critical' in CSM is about prioritising the issue of power in gender relations. Awareness of the relational context of power in gender relations is useful as it begins to answer the question of why men might pursue certain ideals of masculinity, despite the deleterious consequences on their health. Essentially, it is because, as Courtenay (2000: 1833) notes, the very social practices which undermine men's health (assuming their physical and mental health to be strong and invulnerable) allow men to demonstrate manliness and acquire power in sexist and gender-dichotomous societies. Acknowledging the relational context of power suggests that men's lifestyles and attitudes and behaviours to health are embedded in a network of gendered structures and gendered relations in society. Moreover, it draws attention to the embeddedness of men's gendered health practices in broader sets of structural inequalities in society, such as where we live, how we work, support structures that allow us time to cook meals, 'play' and retain our social networks. It is precisely because of the embeddedness of men's health in broader sets of social relations that I believe it is necessary to turn to the broader inequalities in health literature. Thus, the CSM focus on the relational context of power can potentially create the missing link between critical studies of men's health and inequalities in health research.

INTEGRATING THEORIES OF INEQUALITIES IN HEALTH AND CSM

The scientific literature in inequalities in health draws together a literature which examines inequalities at structural (community and global)-level factors as well as at individual-level factors (propensity to smoke, take exercise) into a unified framework. However, there is also much debate within the inequalities literature on the relative importance of precise pathways of inequalities in health and, consequently, the most appropriate points of intervention to address inequalities in health. In order to draw out how CSM theories on men's health might link with the inequalities in health research, I am now going to look at three dominant explanatory pathways: materialist/structuralist, cultural/behavioural and psychosocial. In addition, a life-course approach will be considered alongside these pathways. For each, I address the questions: *What is the explanation?* and *How might the explanation be combined with CSM?*

Materialist/structuralist explanations

What is it?

The materialist explanation may be seen to operate at two of the interrelated levels of influence referred to above – the societal and the individual. At the societal level, the materialist argument, often referred to as the neo-materialist argument, suggests the need to examine how the material conditions of a society – such as investment in health and social care, education and public transport – affect the health of the population of that society. According to this argument, it is strategic investments in neo-material conditions via more equitable distribution of public and private resources that are likely to have the most impact on reducing health inequalities and improving public health in both rich and poor countries in the twenty-first century (Lynch *et al.*, 2000:1203). The materialist/structuralist explanation applied at the individual level refers to how one's access to tangible material goods and conditions (including food, housing, access to amenities, etc.) is associated with exposures that are damaging to, or protective of, health (Adamson *et al.*, 2006: 974). Observed inequalities in health are consistently found to be related to material factors, regardless of which measure is used. The explanation applied to understanding gender inequities in health suggests that gender health inequities are an outcome of inequalities in the socio-economic positions of men and women. Therefore, in so far as there is convergence in men and women's material position, so too should we find convergence in men's and women's health. Indeed, studies that have specifically explored men and women with similar working, social and material circumstances show a reduction in, or absence of, gender-based morbidity (Hall, 1992; Emslie *et al.*, 1999; Umberson *et al.*, 1996; Hraba *et al.*, 1996; Matthews *et al.*, 1999; Arber & Cooper, 1999; Schofield *et al.*, 2000; Bartley, 2004). However, one recent study also (tentatively) disconfirmed the thesis of convergence in gender equality leading to convergence in health status (Backhans *et al.*, 2007).

How might this explanation be combined with CSM?

This explanation has been under-utilised in men's health research because, while socio-economic inequality between men and women can explain women's health disadvantages, it is thought that there is no *socio-economic* theory which can explain men's lower longevity in life expectancy to women (because men are recognised as the more economically and socially advantaged group) (Bird & Rieker, 1999:750). The reduction in the gap in male and female life expectancy (the relative rise in male life expectancy), reported since the 1970s, in advanced capitalist societies in which women show relatively high levels of emancipation, is attributed more to convergence in behaviours, such as increased smoking and drinking among women, which may have been encouraged by economic growth and development (Waldron, 1993; Trovato & Lalu, 1996). The materialist explanation has, however, been invoked in CSM's health research to distinguish *between* men of different socio-economic groups in relation to specific aspects of men's health, such as accessing health care, diet, and health-damaging and health-promoting behaviours (Prättälä *et al.*, 1994; Wilson, 1998; Matheson & Summerfield, 2001; Roos *et al.*, 2001; O'Brien *et al.*, 2005; Robertson, 2006a). Looking at differences in material relations between men is important to teasing out the materialist underpinnings of diversity in men's health status and men's health behaviours and attitudes. However, comparisons with similar groups of women are usually omitted and, consequently, so too is an analysis of the *connections* in the materialist underpinnings of men and women's health (Sabo, 1999; Schofield *et al.*, 2000). Research which does both – examines materialist relations between men as well as between men and women – is required around specific areas of health in order to tease out the interactions between social class and gender in men and women's health.

A further way of opening up the debate between inequalities in health and CSM's health is to think of the materialist/structuralist argument as representing the symbolic power of men over women in society. The hegemony of men, in Hearn's (2004) terms, or masculine domination, in Bourdieu's (2001) terms, includes the symbolic power of masculinity over femininity as well as issues such as wealth and income. The symbolic power of men also fits with the aforementioned materialist/structuralist definition as including social as well as economic capital. As noted earlier, in CSM's health (see in particular, Sabo, 1999; Connell, 2000; Schofield *et al.*, 2000), there is an acknowledgement that it is this very power asymmetry in gender relations which is the underlying motivation for much of men's negative health attitudes and behaviours. Locating the symbolic power of masculinity over femininity as a materialist argument also introduces the interaction between the materialist and cultural/behavioural explanations which will be elaborated below.

Cultural/behavioural explanations

What is it?

This explanation suggests that health inequalities are an outcome of differing cultural attitudes to health and related health behaviours. There are two different models of this explanation – or as Macintyre (1997) suggests, a 'hard' and 'soft' version. The hard version suggests that health-damaging behaviours freely chosen by individuals in different social classes *explain away* social gradients, while the soft version suggests that health-damaging behaviours are differentially distributed across social classes and *contribute to* observed gradients (Macintyre, 1997:727). The hard version owes its origin to the discipline of epidemiology and its concern with the identification of risk factors – most notably unhealthy behaviours and aspects of poor lifestyle management – associated with particular diseases. It suggests that addressing poor health behaviours is 'the most effective way' to prevent disease (Courtenay, 2000). The soft version owes its origin to the broader research on inequalities in health and is linked to the materialist/structuralist explanation which critiques the notion that one can separate individuals' lifestyle choices from individuals' social/cultural and economic milieu. The inequalities in health scholarship argue instead that the empirical focus should be on the context of people's lives, which may provide the 'contextualised rationality' (Williams, 2003) of healthy or unhealthy behavioural patterns (see Lynch *et al.*, 1997 for a review).

The soft version of the behavioural/cultural explanation also differs from the materialist/structuralist explanations outlined above in that it tries to shift the emphasis from income and wealth towards attitudes, values and beliefs, and normative behaviours. However, getting inside the role of culture on health is complex. For example, there is no straightforward connection between attitudes to health and *actual* health behaviours (Bartley, 2004). In Blaxter's (1990) study of lifestyles and health, the strongest anti-smoking views were held by men who smoked. In addition, the inequalities in health literature challenges the idea that 'cultures' (for example, ethnic, feminine, masculine, working-class) are universal and unchanging. Consequently, even though we might assume that cultural processes may be in some way implicated in health outcomes, we cannot assume they will be the same for every member of that cultural group or that cultural norms do not vary in relation to other material and environmental factors.

How might this explanation be combined with CSM?

On the one hand, critical studies of men's health need to be able to acknowledge, where necessary, the relative stability of cultural notions of masculinities (notably hegemonic masculinity) on men's health. On the other hand, they need to avoid essentialising characteristics, such as risk adversity, aggression and competitiveness as 'masculine' or endemic in masculine culture. To this end, CSM's health can contribute to the more sociologically informed – or 'soft' – version of the cultural behavioural explanation in inequalities in health research by highlighting the relative stability of hegemonic concepts of masculinity without relying on cultural reductionism. A key mechanism within CSM for taking culture seriously but avoiding cultural reductionism is prioritising a research focus on diversity in how masculinity and health operate in daily lives between men – and by the same men in relation to different health practices – *and* by relating this diversity to the broader social and economic milieu (see, for example, O'Brien *et al.*, 2005; Robertson, 2006a). A CSM approach equally contrasts with an approach in some health professional literature (as noted earlier) which recommends programmatic ways of dealing with men and men's health issues and, therefore, treats the category of 'men' and 'hegemonic masculinity' as stable and static cultural traits (Seymour-Smith *et al.*, 2002).

CSM's health can also be combined with cultural explanations from the broader inequalities literature by a joint growing interest in an *embodied sociology*. The approach seeks to theorise how relations between the biological and social are experienced through our embodied being in the world (Williams & Bendelow, 1998; Williams *et al.*, 2003). It may be distinguished from the disembodied rational actor in much positivist social science as well as postmodernist theorising (or radically social constructionist models) of the body which deny the biological reality of the body, except as an object formed through situational discourses. Connell (2002: 47–52), for example, writes of *social embodiment*, meaning that bodies have a certain kind of agency and materiality – require food, eat, sleep, are sexually aroused, give birth and die – but are also socially constructed through long and continuous circuits of social structures. The embodied approach opens up more complex understandings of representations of hegemonic masculinities and empirical explorations of how men's bodies are experienced by men in everyday life (Watson, 2000; Klein, 1993; Chapple & Ziebland, 2002; Robertson, 2006b; Oliffe, 2006).

Psychosocial explanation

What is it?

The psychosocial model places primacy on the psychological impact of adverse psychosocial exposures, such as stress, hostility, hopelessness, loss of control or, collectively, the impact of 'misery' on health (Macleod & Davey Smith, 2003: 565). This explanation is also relevant at both the individual and societal or context levels. At the individual level, the explanation purports that stressful social circumstances associated with lower levels of power and social support in the home, the workplace, or society at large, produce emotional responses which, in turn, bring about biological changes which may increase the risk of disease (see Bartley, 2004; Adamson *et al.*, 2006 for an overview). At the societal or contextual level, a major recent hypothesis is derived from the alleged psycho-social effect of the unequal incomes theory (Wilkinson, 1996; 1997; Kawachi *et al.*, 1999). In particular, Wilkinson (1997) and Kawachi *et al.* (1999) have argued that income inequality in societies can create psychosocial reactions which change people's vision of self-esteem and forms of social cohesion or trust (measured in terms of social networks/social involvement) in society. They propose that this, in turn, leads to poorer health via psycho-neuro-endocrine mechanisms as well as through unhealthy coping behaviours, such as excessive drinking and smoking.

However, the field of research – and specifically the unequal incomes thesis – is reported to be at a 'cross-roads' (Lynch & Davey Smith, 2002; Pearce & Davey Smith, 2003; Lynch et al., 2004). In a recent major review of studies on income inequality and health, Lynch et al. (2004) concluded that there is some evidence to support the thesis at the state level in the United States but not as a generalisable determinant of health in Western developed countries. More broadly in relation to the psychosocial thesis, some authors (notably, Shaw et al., 1999, Lynch et al., 2001; Macleod and Davey Smith, 2003; Lynch et al., 2004, Adamson et al., 2006), while acknowledging that 'misery' and poverty may be interrelated, have contested the primacy of the psychological aetiological pathway implied in the psychosocial explanation. Instead, they assert that health differences are primarily related to the lifetime material well-being of social groups, including factors such as access to good quality accommodation, diet, and leisure pursuits, and not to the psychological effects of positions within hierarchies.

How might this explanation be combined with CSM?

The debate on the potential impact of psychosocial pathways on health is one of the most controversial debates in inequalities in health research. However, the ways in which psychosocial pathways may be gendered and, particularly, the way masculinities are implicated in these psychosocial pathways is neglected. At the individual level, the psychosocial hypothesis may be usefully combined with theories of protest masculinity from CSM (Connell, 1995). The combined explanation applied to men's health would propose that the effect on men of being economically and socially unequal (to other men especially, and possibly also to some women) generates psychological feelings of poor self-esteem related to inequality which can itself be directly health-damaging. Further, feelings of economic and social inequality may lead some men to engage in extreme macho behaviours in order to regain social status through appealing to hierarchies of masculinity rather than hierarchies of social class (see Canaan, 1996; O' Brien *et al.*, 2005). The added value to men's health research of incorporating the psychosocial explanation is to look at the psychosocial effects of positions in hierarchies (class, gender ethnic) simultaneously, such that the impact of masculinities may be seen in relation to class and ethnicity. In addition, it is to theorise some men's 'negative health behaviours' as a form of agency to overcome other types of inequalities which may also account for the relative obduracy of negative health behaviours amongst some groups of men.

A life-course approach to understanding inequalities in health

What is it?

A life-course approach to understanding inequalities in health is not necessarily a *different* explanation to those already discussed. Rather, a life-course approach incorporates elements of the materialist, behavioural and psychosocial pathways but lengthens the causal chain of these explanations. The life-course explanation suggests that health status at any given age for a given birth cohort reflects not only contemporary conditions, but embodiment of prior life conditions from *in utero* onwards (Kawachi *et al.*, 2002:650). The life-course approach incorporates a range of conceptual models to capture these temporal relationships. The three models commonly identified are critical period models, pathway models and accumulation models. The models may be seen as being broadly complementary in that all three models direct attention to biographies of disadvantage (Graham, 2002: 2008). A *critical period model* (also known as latent effects or latency model) (Ben-Shlomo & Kuh, 2002; Kawachi *et al.*, 2002) suggests that diseases which make a greater contribution to the socio-economic gradient in health have their origins in critical periods of development. Critical period models tend to focus on the contribution of early life adversity, highlighting embryonic, infant and childhood periods (such as Barker's foetal programming hypothesis [Barker, 1999]) as major influences on disease risk in adulthood

(Graham, 2002:2008). The *pathway model* focuses on how early life environment sets individuals onto life trajectories which have implications for health (for example, how childhood disadvantage may restrict educational opportunities which may in turn restrict employment opportunities and health-related behaviours in later life). The *accumulation* or cumulative effects model suggests that the intensity or duration of exposure to unfavourable environments at different life stages has a cumulative or 'chain' adverse effect on health. According to this model, poor circumstances throughout life confer the greatest risk of poor health in adulthood (Graham, 2002: 2008). Many of the studies in this field have shown that it is the cumulative effect over time of low income in combination with other indicators of poverty, such as low birth weight, poor educational attainment and poor employment conditions, which account for inequalities in health (see Shaw *et al.*, 1999; Lynch *et al.*, 2001; Graham, 2002). However, according to this model, poor circumstances at one stage in life can be mitigated by better circumstances earlier or later in life (Graham, 2002: 2008).

How might this explanation be combined with CSM?

There has been quite a large body of work going back some time, on differences in women's health in relation to what might be called points in the life course, for example, differences in women's health in relation to marital status, age of children, or movement in and out of the labour force (see Bartley, 2004: ch. 9; Arber & Cooper, 1999 for overviews of this research). By contrast, there has been comparatively little qualitative research identifying how key life moments/transition points may impact on men's health and well-being either in a positive or negative way (for some exceptions, see Ferketich & Mercer, 1989; Watson, 2000; Robertson, 2003; Bartlett, 2004). In addition, there is a need to take an explicit life-course approach to this work which could strengthen CSM's health-specific focus on understanding masculinities and health by exploring the ways cultural constructions of hegemonic masculinity are subject to change over time. The life-course approach suggests that there is a need to conduct longitudinal panel studies in qualitative research which could look in greater depth at the contextualised *cumulative* effect of these events/milestones on gendered health patterns. Hence, there is a need for prospective longitudinal research designs which may involve researching parental accounts of foetal and child health initially until consent may be obtained to interview/collect diaries from young boys and adults at regular intervals throughout their lives. Alternatively, the retrospective life-course design is easier to implement (such as Oliffe, 2007). Also, in research on African men's health, in particular, there has been a welcome attempt to unravel the antecedents of contemporary masculinities in the historical gendered cultural politics through which they have been produced, and to study their impact on men's health, especially men's sexual health behaviours in the context of HIV/AIDS (Hunter, 2005; Simpson, 2005).

CONCLUSION

To date, the major gap in male and female mortality in the Western world has been attributed to behavioural differences between men and women (Stanistreet *et al.*, 2005). In particular, studies of men's health have focused on the role of 'hegemonic masculinities' in influencing men's health behaviours and men's health status. By contrast, the inequalities literature is based upon seeing health as an outcome of the complex interplay of a range of factors associated with the circumstances under which people live out their lives, but has largely neglected men's health. This chapter has been about developing some intellectual cohesion between research on men, masculinities and health and the broader inequalities in health literature. I have argued that making this link relies first and foremost on a keener reading of *critical studies on men* rather than men's studies. The former is the more sociologically and feminist-grounded wing of the men and masculinities literature and can, therefore, be more easily forged with the duality of structure and agency, which is a feature of the explanatory models of inequalities in health research. I have also sought to demonstrate how the literature on men and masculinities may be incorporated into an inequalities-in-health explanatory framework in order to more fully explain men's health. Combining the literatures suggests the need to study concurrently the impact of materialist/structural cultural/behavioural, psychosocial factors in the context of a life-course approach in understanding men's health. The implication of this chapter is that future studies of men's health, as well as health promotion interventions for men, should take on board the wider range of health-determinant variables that is made possible by drawing from a combined explanatory framework.

REFERENCES

Adamson, J.A., Ebrahim, S. & Hunt, K. (2006) The psychosocial versus material hypothesis to explain observed inequality in disability among older adults: data from the West of Scotland Twenty-07 Study. *Journal of Epidemiology and Community Health*, 60, 974–80.

Arber, S. & Cooper, H. (1999) Gender differences in health in later life: the new paradox? *Social Science & Medicine*, 48(1), 61–76.

Backhans, M.C., Lundberg, M. & Månsdotter, A. (2007) Does increased gender equality lead to a convergence of health outcomes for men and women? A study of Swedish municipalities. *Social Science & Medicine*, 64, 1892–1903.

Barker, D.J.P. (1999) Foetal programming and public health. In P.M.S. O'Brien, T. Wheelar & D.J.P. Barker (eds), *Foetal Programming: Influences on Development and Disease in Later Life*. London: Royal College of Obstetricians and Gynaecologists, p. 3.

Bartlett, E. (2004) The effects of fatherhood on the health of men: a review of the literature. *Journal of Men's Health and Gender*, 1 (2–3),159–69.

Bartley, M. (2004) *Health Inequality: An Introduction to Theories, Concepts and Methods*. Cambridge: Polity.

Ben-Shlomo, Y. & Kuh, D. (2002) A life course approach to chronic disease epidemiology: conceptual models, empirical challenges and interdisciplinary perspectives. *International Journal of Epidemiology*, 31, 285–93.

Bird, C.E. & Rieker, P.P. (1999) Gender matters: an integrated model for understanding men's and women's health. *Social Science & Medicine*, 48, 745–55.

Blaxter, M. (1990) *Health and Lifestyles*. London: Tavistock.

Bly, R. (1990) *Iron John*. New York: Addison-Wesley.

Bourdieu, P. (2001) *Masculine Domination*. Cambridge: Polity.

Canaan, J. (1996) One thing leads to another: drinking, fighting and working-class masculinities. In M. Mac an Ghaill (ed.), *Understanding Masculinities*. Buckingham: Open University Press, pp. 114–25.

Carrigan, T., Connell, R.W. & Lee, J. 1985. Toward a new sociology of masculinity. *Theory and Society*, 14(5), 551–604.

Chapple, A. & Ziebland, S. (2002) Prostate cancer: embodied experience and perceptions of masculinity. *Sociology of Health & Illness*, 24(6), 820–41.

Coleman, C. & Lohan, M. (forthcoming) Men who have sex with men and partner notification in Ireland: beyond binary dualisms of gender and health care. *Current Sociology*.

Connell, R.W. (1995) *Masculinities*. Cambridge: Polity.

Connell, R.W. (2000) *The Men and the Boys*. Cambridge: Polity.

Connell, R. (2002) *Gender*. Cambridge: Polity.

Connell, R. W. & Messerschmidt, J. W. (2005) Hegemonic masculinity rethinking the concept. *Gender & Society*, 19(6), 829–59.

Connell, R.W., Schofield, T., Walker, L., Wood, J., Butland, D., Fischer, J. & Bowyer, J. (1999) *Men's Health: A Research Agenda and Background Report*. Canberra: Commonwealth Department of Health and Aged Care.

Courtenay, W.H. (2000) Constructions of masculinity and their influence on men's well-being: a theory of gender and health. *Social Science & Medicine*, 50(10), 1385–401.

Doyal, L. (2000) Gender equity in health: debates and dilemmas. *Social Science & Medicine*, 51(6), 931–9.

Emslie C., Hunt K. & Macintyre S. (1999) Problematizing gender, work and health: the relationship between gender, occupational grade, working conditions and minor morbidity in full-time bank employees. *Social Science & Medicine*, 48(1), 33–48.

Faludi, S. (1999) *Stiffed: The Betrayal of the Modern Man*. London: Chatto & Windus.

Farrell, W. (1993) *The Myth of Male Power: Why Men are the Disposable Sex*. New York: Simon & Schuster.

Ferketich, S.L. & Mercer, M.T. (1989) Men's health status during pregnancy and early fatherhood. *Research in Nursing and Health*, 12, 137–48.

Gough, B. (2006) Try to be healthy, but don't forgo your masculinity: deconstructing men's health discourse in the media. *Social Science & Medicine*, 63, 2476–88.

Graham, H. (2002) Building an inter-disciplinary science of health inequalities: the example of life-course research. *Social Science & Medicine*, 55(11), 2006–16.

Hall, E.M. (1992) Double exposure: the combined impact of home and work environments on psychosomatic strain in Swedish women and men. *International Journal of Health Services*, 22(2), 239–60.

Hearn, J. (2004) From hegemonic masculinity to the hegemony of men. *Feminist Theory*, 5(1), 97–120.

Hearn, J. & Morgan, D. (eds) (1990) *Men, Masculinities and Social Theory*. London and New York: Unwin Hyman and Routledge.

Hraba, J., Lorenz, F., Lee, G. & Pechachova, Z. (1996) Gender differences in health: evidence from the Czech Republic. *Social Science & Medicine*, 43(7), 1143–51.

Hunter, M. (2005) Cultural politics and masculinities: multiple-partners in historical perspective in KwaZulu-Natal. *Culture, Health & Sexuality*, 7(4), 389–403.

Kawachi, I., Kennedy, B.P. & Wilkinson, R.G. (eds) (1999) *The Society and Population Health Reader: Vol. 1, Income Inequality and Health*. New York: New Press.

Kawachi, I., Subramanian, S.V. & Almeida-Filho, N. (2002) A glossary for health inequalities. *Journal of Epidemiology and Community Health*, 56(9), 647–52.

Kegan Gardiner, J. (2005) Men, masculinities and feminist theory. In M.S. Kimmel, J. Hearn & R.W. Connell (eds) (2005) *Handbook of Studies on Men and Masculinities*. London: Sage, pp. 35–50.

Kimmel, M. (ed.) (1987). *Changing Men: New Directions in Research on Men and Masculinity*. Newbury Park, CA: Sage.

Kimmel, M.S., Hearn, J. & Connell, R.W. (2005) *Handbook of Studies on Men and Masculinities*. London: Sage.

Klein, A. (1993) *Little Big Men: Bodybuilding Subculture and Gender Construction*. Albany: State University Press of New York Press.

Lynch, J. & Davey-Smith, G. (2002) Commentary: income inequality and health: the end of the story. *International Journal of Epidemiology*, 31(3), 549–51.

Lynch, J., Davey-Smith, G., Harper, S., Hillemeier, M., Ross, N., Kaplan, G.A. & Wolfson, M. (2004) Is income inequality a determinant of population health? Part 1. A systematic review. *Milbank Quarterly*, 82(1), 5–99.

Lynch, J.W., Davey-Smith, G., Hillemeier, M., Shaw, M., Raghunathan, T. & Kaplan, G. (2001) Income inequality, the psychosocial environment and health: comparisons of wealthy nations. *Lancet*, 358(9277), 194–200.

Lynch, J.W., Davey-Smith, G., Kaplan, G. & House, J. (2000) Income inequality and mortality: importance to health of individual income, psychosocial environment or material conditions. *British Medical Journal*, 320, 1200–4.

Lynch, J.W., Kaplan, G.A. & Salonen, J.T. (1997) Why do poor people behave poorly? Variation in adult health behaviours and psychosocial characteristics by stages of socioeconomic lifecourse. *Social Science & Medicine*, 44(6), 809–19.

Macintyre, S. (1997) The black report and beyond: what are the issues? *Social Science & Medicine*, 44(6), 723–45.

Macleod, J. & Davey Smith, G. (2003) Psychosocial factors and public health: a suitable case for treatment? *Journal of Epidemiology and Community Health*, 57: 565–70.

Matheson, J. & Summerfield, C. (2001) *Social Focus on Men*. London: Stationery Office.

Matthews S., Manor O. & Power C. (1999) Social inequalities in health: are there gender differences? *Social Science & Medicine*, 48(1), 49–60.

Moynihan, C. (1998) Theories in health care and research: theories of masculinity. *British Medical Journal*, 317, 1072–5.

O'Brien, R., Hunt, K. & Hart, G. (2005) 'It's caveman stuff, but that is to a certain extent how guys still operate': men's accounts of masculinity and help-seeking. *Social Science & Medicine*, 61(3), 503–16.

Oliffe, J. L. (2006) Embodied masculinity and androgen deprivation therapy. *Sociology of Health & Illness*, 28(4), 410–32.

Oliffe, J. L. (2007) Health behaviors, prostate cancer and masculinities: a life course perspective. In *Men and Masculinities*. Advance online publication. Retrieved 21 January 2008.

Pearce, N. & Davey Smith, G. (2003) Is social capital the key to inequalities in health? *American Journal of Public Health*, 93(1), 122–9.

Phillips, M. (1999) *The Sex-Change Society: Feminised Britain and the Neutered Male*. London: Social Market Foundation.

Prättälä, R., Karisto, A. & Berg, M.A. (1994) Consistency and variation in unhealthy behaviour among Finish men, 1982–1990. *Social Science & Medicine*, 39(1), 53–64.

Robertson, S. (2003) 'If I let a goal in, I'll get beat up': contradictions in masculinity sport and health. *Health Education Research*, 18(6), 706–16.

Robertson, S. (2006a) 'Not living life in too much of an excess': lay men understanding health and well-being. *Health*, 10(2), 175–89.

Robertson, S. (2006b) 'I've been like a coiled spring this last week': embodied masculinity and health. *Sociology of Health & Illness*, 28(4), 433–56.

Robertson S. & Williamson, P. (2005) Men and health promotion in the UK: ten years further on? *Health Education Journal*, 64(4), 293–301.

Roos, G., Prättälä, R. & Koski, K. (2001) Men, masculinity and food: interviews with Finnish carpenters and engineers. *Appetite*, 37(1), 47–56.

Sabo, D. (1999) *Understanding Men's Health: A Relational and Gender Sensitive Approach.* Harvard Centre for Population and Development Studies: Working Paper Series, No. 99.14.

Sabo, D. & Gordon, D.F. (eds) *Men's Health and Illness: Gender, Power and the Body.* Thousand Oaks, CA: Sage.

Saltonstall, R. (1993) Healthy bodies, social bodies: men's and women's concepts and practices of health in everyday life. *Social Science & Medicine*, 36(1): 7–14.

Schofield, T., Connell, R., Walker, L., Wood, J. & Butland, D. (2000) Understanding men's health and illness: a gender-relations approach to policy, research and practice. *Journal of American College Health*, 48(6), 247–55.

Segal, L. (1990). *Slow Motion: Changing Masculinities, Changing Men.* London: Virago and Rutgers University Press.

Seymour-Smith, S. Wetherell, M. and Phoenix, A. (2002) 'My wife ordered me to come!' A discursive analysis of doctors' and nurses' accounts of men's use of General Practitioners. *Journal of Health Psychology*, 7, 253–66.

Shaw, M., Dorling, D, Gordon, D. & Davey-Smith, G. (1999) *The Widening Gap: Health Inequalities and Policy in Britain.* Bristol: Policy Press.

Simpson, A. (2005) Sons and fathers/boys to men in the time of AIDS: learning masculinity in Zambia. *Journal of South African Studies*, 31(3), 569–86.

Stanistreet, D., Bambra, C. & Scott-Samuel, A. (2005) Is patriarchy the source of men's higher mortality? *Journal of Epidemiology and Community Health*, 59, 873–6.

Trovato, F. & Lalu, N. (1996). Narrowing sex differentials in life expectancy in the industrialized world: early 1970s to early 1990s. *Social Biology*, 43(1–2): 20–37.

Tsuchiya, A. & Williams, A. (2005) A 'fair innings' between the sexes: are men being treated inequitably? *Social Science & Medicine,* 60(2), 277–86.

Umberson, J.D., Chen, M. D., House, J.S., Hopkins, K. & Slater, E. (1996) The effect of social relationships on psychological well-being. Are men and women really so different? *American Sociological Review*, 61(5), 837–57.

Waldron, I. (1991) Patterns and causes of gender differences in smoking. *Social Science & Medicine*, 32: 989–1005.

Watson, J. (2000) *Male Bodies: Health Culture and Identity.* Buckingham: Open University Press.

White, A. (2001) How men respond to illness. *Men's Health Journal,* 1(1),18–19.

White, A. & Cash, K. (2004) The state of men's health in Western Europe, *Journal of Men's Health & Gender,* 1(1), 60–6.

White, A. & Johnson, M. (2000) Men making sense of their chest pain – niggles, doubts and denials. *Journal of Clinical Nursing,* 9, 534–41.

Whitehead, S.M. (2002) *Men and Masculinities.* Cambridge: Polity.

Wilkinson, R.G. (1996) *Unhealthy Societies: The Afflictions of Inequality.* London: Routledge.

Wilkinson, R.G. (1997) Socio-economic determinants of health. Health inequalities: Relative or absolute material standards? *British Medical Journal,* 314(7080): 591–5.

Williams, G. (2003) The determinants of health: structure, context and agency. *Sociology of Health and Illness,* 25 (Silver Anniversary Issue): 131–54.

Williams, S.J. & Bendelow, G. (1998) *The Lived Body: Sociological Themes, Embodied Issues.* London: Routledge.

Wilson, A. (1998) Getting help. In T. O'Dowd & D. Jewell (eds), *Men's Health.* Oxford: Oxford University Press, pp. 273–271.

2 A GRAND ILLUSION: MASCULINITY, 'PASSING' AND MEN'S HEALTH

David Buchbinder

INTRODUCTION

What do Superman, Spider-Man and the Hulk have in common, aside from enjoying the status of superheroes and displaying the inclination to fight crime and evil? This may seem an odd question with which to begin a chapter included in a volume on men's health. Moreover, in the context of several decades of public concern and media reports about men's health – for example, increasing levels of obesity, the excessive use of alcohol, risk-taking practices, violent behaviour, and cardiovascular and pulmonary problems caused by abuse of the body, as well as men's reluctance to present to a health professional earlier rather than later – this question may also seem irrelevant. It is, however, a pertinent one for a discussion that adopts a cultural studies approach.

Where most writing on men's health draws on largely empirical data within a medical, sociological or anthropological frame, cultural studies looks to the culture itself and the 'texts' it produces, whether these are material artefacts or cultural and social practices, in order to explore the way these texts represent a particular object of examination. Such representations are not merely neutral reflections of what 'really' goes on in the culture. Rather, they encode ideological imperatives and discursive constellations concerning the ways people act and 'think' themselves; and they help to naturalise these so that they seem quite unexceptionable – indeed, logical and inevitable – to people in the culture. Accordingly, therefore, textual representations in media such as film, television and advertising, as well as in literature and art, constitute for the cultural studies scholar the relevant field of research and yield the data that form the empirical material on which to base findings and conclusions.

Much of the concern expressed, especially in the popular media but also in professional publications, over the past two or three decades about men's health has tended to assume a relatively local and isolatable cause for issues in this area. At the level of the individual, men's behaviours are often attributed to 'lifestyle choices', so that practices with negative or deleterious consequences for a man's health are understood as grounded in decisions made by the individual male, who is then tacitly or explicitly responsible for his behaviour and its effects on his well-being. Thus, for example,[1] Tamara McLean, in an article dated 11 April 2008 and published on the news.com.au website, a division of Rupert Murdoch's News Corporation, begins with the statement: 'The majority of Australian men are fat but only half of them know it, according to new research showing an alarming number are in denial about their weight' (McLean, 2008). Similarly, Robyn Riley, in her article of 23 March 2008, 'Men's Health: A National Scandal', published in the *Herald Sun* (another Murdoch paper, available on heraldsun.com.au), opines that 'Men are apathetic about their health and women brush the problem aside, complaining it should not be up to them to make their blokes see a doctor' (Riley, 2008). Even *NSW Health*, a website owned by the New South Wales Government Department of Health, is not exempt from implicit assumptions about men's individual and localised responsibilities for health. Although it does invoke broader, contextual and environmental influences on men's health – for instance: 'For adult men, a major influence on health is the workplace. For men who are unemployed, health impacts may differ. There are also many men for whom the loss, grief and other difficulties involved with relationship breakdown lead to lingering health issues. Some research suggests the need to focus interventions (such as counselling) at the time of separation' and 'Things like work and income interact with ethnicity, sexual and cultural identity and age to influence men's health status' – there are nonetheless implications that individual males fail to deal adequately and effectively with such issues as grief; while the statement that 'Older men may find their role changing from one of breadwinner to homemaker, as one in three carers over the age of 60 is male. But many may lack the skills required for cooking a nutritious meal and arranging social interaction', despite its careful phrasing, implies that the behaviours, practices and attitudes of the individual man may be the source and cause of his own ill health (New South Wales Department of Health, 2001: 2).

Alternatively, other, more general causes may be invoked as having negative impacts on men's health. For example, changes in the workplace and in marriage and family profile and dynamics have been largely laid at the door of feminism and the women's movements from the 1970s onward. The greater social and economic independence of women, together with the higher profile of women in business organisations, so the story goes, has resulted in the diminution of men's role as providers, and in greater competition for employment and position, competition which, from some perspectives, has been seen as predetermined in favour of women and therefore as detrimental to men. Feminism and changes in social structures and dynamics have been blamed also for the problem of boys in school: their behaviours and attitudes and their failure to perform up to a required standard are seen as caused by boys' confusion as to how they are to perform their gender roles as men in a world increasingly dominated by women who have come to rely less upon men.[2] The increasing social openness and tolerance of gay, lesbian and queer subjectivities and 'lifestyles' have likewise been adduced as contributing to a so-called crisis in masculinity in the late twentieth and early twenty-first centuries.[3] Where masculinity once seemed simply and naturally definable in terms of appropriateness of sex (women were ineligible because they were female) and of sexuality (homosexual men were ineligible because they desired other men), now gender and the requirements it imposes on individuals have come to seem more complicated, slippery and difficult.

Historical moments, too, have been made to bear the blame for the problems that men face, and which have had impact on their health behaviours and practices. For instance, the trend in business in the late 1980s and 1990s to 'downsize' and 'rationalise' meant that many males lost their jobs; and, because since the Industrial Revolution in the late eighteenth century masculinity has been defined strongly in terms of a man's capacity to find employment and to support himself and his family, this had significant consequences for men's health, in terms of an increase in diagnosed depression, suicide rates and the like. Moreover, feminism and the women's movements could again be held responsible here: more women in the workforce meant that fewer jobs were available to men, and positive discrimination policies in favour of women made many men feel that they were being made the scapegoats for bad gender policies on the part of the corporations and organisations that had employed them and which now capitulated to women's demands.[4]

What is not always explored and examined as a key factor in the statistics regarding men's health, however, is the way that gender itself and gender behaviours are constructed in the culture, and how these may result in the sorts of practices that are identified as imperilling men's health. Masculinity is formed within a patriarchal discourse of gender; and while this has historically both privileged and benefited men, it has by its very nature positioned men in certain ways, and has exerted a variety of pressures upon them. As I have argued elsewhere (see Buchbinder, 1994: 32–8), this discourse actually defines masculinity as a status rather than a quality or set of qualities, and requires that such status be attained through competition with other males in a wide spectrum of social situations and structures, ranging from the amicable contests engaged in by friends (for instance, competition in an individual's capacity to hold his liquor or to 'score' sexually with women) to open rivalry (for instance, in seeking promotion in an organisation). Masculinity as status is therefore conferred upon the individual man by other men,[5] *who equally have the authority to rescind it*. That this is the case can be discerned in terms of the opprobrium – 'You run like a girl', 'Poofter!' – meted out by men to other males, even in relatively friendly social situations.

Such a state of affairs necessitates, for the individual male, that his quest for status as fully masculine take place within a context of competition with precisely those other males who can bestow or withhold a man's title to masculinity. Accordingly, then, a man's sense of himself as a fully masculine subject is rendered still more unstable by the awareness, however tentative or vague, of the perpetual contingency or provisionality of his status as masculine; and of the capacity of other men to withdraw or withhold it from him. As a result, a fundamental insecurity and radical anxiety must underlie even the most macho of masculine performances by individual men. That insecurity and anxiety are then likely to lead in turn to the kinds of manifest, symptomatic behaviours on which health professionals and official health policies tend to focus, such as excessive alcohol consumption or the reluctance to reveal vulnerability, together with a complementary inclination toward risk-taking practices, and the internalisation and subsequent repression of emotional response to external events and situations. It is important there- fore to develop understandings of the discursive structuring and dynamics of masculinity as a particular configuration within the discourse of gender, and to include an approach to men's health issues from that perspective, rather than seeing those issues sim- ply as the consequence of individual men's choices, and their action or failure to take action.

Drawing on the work of the linguists John Searle and J.L. Austin, Judith Butler (1993) proposes in *Bodies That Matter: On the Discursive Limits of 'Sex'* that gender, far from being a sim- ple and natural assignment of behaviour based on genital con- figuration, is in fact *performative*. Searle and Austin suggest that certain speech acts do what they say: for example, the *saying* of a promise is the *undertaking* of the promise:

> *Performative acts are forms of authoritative speech: most performatives, for instance, are statements that, in the uttering, also perform a certain action and exercise a binding power. Implicated in a network of authorization and punish- ment, performatives tend to include legal sentences, baptisms, inaugurations, declarations of ownership, statements which not only perform an action, but confer a binding power on the action performed. If the power of discourse to produce that which it names is linked with the question of performativity, then the performative is one domain in which power acts as discourse.*
>
> *(Butler, 1993: 225)*

Gendered behaviour is performative, suggests Butler, not because of an inevitable connection between anatomical sex and gendered behaviour, but because the subject manifesting that behaviour *wishes to be taken as belonging to* a particular gender. We can think of this as an 'as if' scenario: the individual subject acts *as if* 'she' or 'he' belonged to a particular gender category.

Butler argues further that, precisely because the relationship of sex to gender is thus tenuous and unstable, the culture exerts pressure on its members constantly to repeat or 'cite' the gen- der behaviour demanded of their respective sex: 'In the first instance, performativity must be understood not as a singular or deliberate "act," but, rather, as the reiterative and citational practice by which discourse produces the effects that it names' (Butler 1993: 2).

There is, however, a certain shiftiness in the discourse of gender: if, as Butler argues, gender is indeed performative, nonetheless the discourse presents it – and exerts pressure for it to be understood – as *constative*; that is, as making statements about the world that are both descriptive and true. It is in this gap between gender behaviour as performative and gender behaviour as constative that we all play out our roles as men or women. One might argue, then, following Butler, that macho masculinity is the *emphatic* citation of gender, intended to dispel any doubts about the male subject's gender claim not only for others but also – and especially – for himself. Normative masculinity, then, may be understood as *masculinity proficiently performed*. This includes, of course, the individual man's sense of well-being, since the discourse of traditional masculinity tends to define ill health as, in some measure, feminising; but also his ability to demonstrate the so-called manly virtues, such as stoicism, physical and mental strength, fortitude, courage, and so on, many of which are integral to the calculus of power by which a patriarchal system operates. Indeed, the failure convincingly to display any of these traits is likely to produce in the individual male a sense – whether physical or psychological – of a failure also to be fully a man, which in turn may have serious consequences for that individual's physical and/or mental health.

So, to return to my opening question, what *do* Superman, Spider-Man, the Hulk and a number of other superheroes have in common? The answer is: they have, for the most part, extraordinarily ordinary alter egos. Indeed, one might go so far as to say that those alter egos, however good-looking, intelligent, affable, honest and worthy, are presented as inadequately or incompetently masculine in the performative sense, according to the criteria that govern the culture's understanding of an ideal masculinity. Clark Kent, Peter Parker and David Banner (the 'others' to Superman, Spider-Man and the Hulk) seem at various times, at least to those around them, to be physically weak, awkward, cowardly, disengaged, focused on the mundane rather than the heroic, even geeky or nerdish. Indeed, geekiness seems to be constructed as the polar opposite of 'real' masculinity: perceived as physically unattractive, lacking in true manly courage and bravado, and hence frequently feminised, the geek may be ostracised, ridiculed, vilified and otherwise exiled to the margins of the masculine and hence also of the social world.[6]

The comic books and movies featuring these superheroes and their alternate identities have traditionally been aimed chiefly at young male audiences. We may infer, therefore, that there is a message aimed at this readership in these narratives about masculinity and the behaviours appropriate to it. For these readers, then, 'true' or 'real' masculinity is represented as manifested in a certain charisma, better than average looks, a strong and imposing physique, the capacity for courageous, even daring action, and a stoic attitude, all liberally laced with a strong sense of the social good and with a pronounced strain of ethical rectitude, mitigated by compassion. While the alter ego may be equally concerned with the social good and with the right ethical sense, he is usually represented as too timorous, hesitant and ineffectual to be classified with the 'real' masculine figure, the superhero proper. Accordingly, the young male reader is invited to align the superhero with other heroic manly types who manifest boldness, strength and decisiveness. Importantly, these qualities may also be read as signalling the potential presence of male aggressiveness and violence, understood as inherent in the male subject – and made explicit in the figure of the Hulk, as well as in cases where the superhero turns bad, as, for example, in *Spider-Man 3* – but here domesticated and brought into the service of the common social good and all that this implies, in terms of a culturally acceptable ethics and morality.

The superhero, moreover, exerts a physical appeal that may be overtly or covertly sexual. Not only is the superhero conventionally handsome – the Hulk here is the exception that proves the rule – but the superhero costume is traditionally tight-fitting and form-revealing. However, lest the young male reader's eye be drawn to the superhero's crotch – the male genitals being an object culturally prohibited in a social patriarchal order to both the male gaze and male desire – the latter is modestly concealed beneath a garment that strongly resembles men's underpants; yet, ironically, that concealment actually *solicits* the eye's attention to the contrast between the often gaudy costume and the differently coloured garment of modesty. Despite the cultural prohibition, the male reader is thus invited to become aware of and to contemplate the hero's super-genitals. The anxiety that permeates a patriarchal culture about male–male desire and the homoerotic is therefore always already inscribed into the superhero narrative, a genre which, it seems, both encourages homoerotic desire at the same time as it seeks to avert and forbid it.

Indeed, it may be said that masculinity – in our culture at least – is constructed around a constellation of anxieties which are generated by the concern provoked by a key duality: is a proper man one who conforms to the standards of an idealised 'true' masculinity, as signified by the characteristic traits of the superhero, or one who embodies, rather, more ordinary traits, which in comparison may be perceived as signalling a less proficiently performed masculinity? I propose to call this latter figure the *schlemiel*. The word derives from Yiddish, the language of diasporic European Jewry, and signifies a comic figure, clumsy, hapless, destined to be not only a social but also a cosmic fool. There are many thumbnail definitions and sketches of the schlemiel: for instance, in his series of definitions, Leo Rosten quotes the Yiddish saying that 'The shlemiel [*sic*] falls on his back and breaks his nose' (1971: 352).[7] The schlemiel, then, represents a less than ideal masculinity; and in the competitive dynamic of patriarchal masculinity he generally acquires the status only of the also-ran. In the cultural imaginary of gender and specifically of masculinity, then, the male subject is offered a radical and reductive choice between the gender and behavioural options that I am calling the superhero and the schlemiel: his behaviour as a man will assign him to one or the other category.[8]

The tensions occasioned by this polarisation and the imposed assignment of the individual male to one of the classes of the masculine find an answering echo in the social behaviour of men, and the practices of masculinity that they then adopt. Because it is the superhero figure who attracts the plaudits, admiration and respect of men, individual males strive to find ways in which to qualify for entry into this category, ways which will often have implications for the health or otherwise of those men. For example, the effort to reproduce within their own bodies the idealised physique of the superhero and also, by implication (because such a physique functions as a sign of these), the other attributed qualities and traits of the superhero, can lead to an obsession with body and body image, and even to eating disorders, as well as the ingestion of such drugs as steroids,[9] while the fear of being relegated to the schlemiel camp can encourage other risky behaviours.

The discourse of gender moreover constructs in the super-hero story a further narrative about masculinity in which the superhero as central character is represented as the 'real' iden-tity, while the schlemiel alter ego functions merely as the dispos-able, and hence inauthentic, cover or disguise for that identity. Yet clearly, in the terms of that narrative, superhero and schle-miel are indissociably connected: not only do both inhabit the same body (despite any physiological changes required, as in the case of the Hulk, to transform from alter ego to superhero) but *each requires the other in order to signify at all*. But what if it is the schlemiel who represents the actual default masculinity – the masculinity of day-to-day reality – while the superhero charac-ter operates merely as his mask? If so, the superhero persona is deployed simply in order to allow the individual (normally schle-miel) male to 'pass' as fully and self-evidently masculine.

Passing as both a social behaviour and political stratagem or ruse is generally taken to operate chiefly in the areas of race and sexuality, so that, for example, black may pass for white or gay for straight. However, as Brooke Kroeger observes, 'There is gen-der passing, class passing, and age passing ... There is even what is erroneously termed "reverse passing", as in straight for gay or white for black, along with dozens of acts of racial, ethnic, and national claim or camouflage' (2003: 5). The notion of passing, therefore, may be understood to have a much wider set of appli-cations and meanings than is generally assumed.

Of the performativity of gender Butler comments, 'this act is not primarily theatrical' (1993: 12); yet, if gender is performa-tive, by its nature it is at the very least spectacular, in the sense that it requires an audience of some kind. Here Michel Foucault's application of Jeremy Bentham's notion of the panopticon is both pertinent and useful. Bentham imagined a prison consist-ing of a many-tiered ring of cells open to a central tower whose windows allowed the guards to observe the prisoners in the cells but which prevented the prisoners from knowing whether and when they were being observed. As a consequence, Foucault notes, the prisoners would be driven to keep themselves under surveillance, since they could never be certain if their behaviour was being officially surveilled or not (1979: 200–209). Similarly, the discourse of gender functions not only to induce us to ensure that those around us conform to the dictates of the discourse, but also to make certain that we ourselves conform. Thus, even in our most solitary moments we continue to perform our discursively assigned gender script as though there were an invisible audience observing us. That is, we seek always to pass as the appropriate gender identity, *even when alone*.

Linda Schlossberg argues that

> *Theories and practices of identity and subject formation in Western culture are largely structured around a logic of visibility, whether in the service of science (Victorian physiognomy), psychoanalysis (Lacan's mirror stage), or philosophy (Foucault's reading of the Panopticon). At the most basic level, we are subjects constituted by visions of ourselves and others, and we trust that our ability to see and read carries with it a certain degree of epistemological certainty ... because of this seemingly intimate relationship between the visual and the known, passing becomes a highly charged site for anxieties regarding visibility, invisibility, classification, and social demarcation.*
>
> *(2001: 1)*

The 'male mastery over masculinity' (Ullman, 2001: 203) thus depends on its visibility, and the nature of that visibility, to others.

In her article '"It Takes One to Know One": Passing and Communities of Common Interest', Amy Robinson identifies passing as a form of duping, citing Elin Diamond's formulation, a 'realism without truth' (Robinson, 1994: 728). She suggests that for a subject's passing to be detected, 'Three participants – the passer, the dupe, and a representative of the in-group – enact a complex narrative scenario in which a successful pass is performed in the presence of a literate member of the in-group' (p. 723). By 'in-group' Robinson means the group out of which the passer seeks to pass, but whose members may be able to recognise the strategies of passing employed by the passer – hence the main title of her article. The 'dupe' is a member of the (often dominant) group into which the passer seeks to pass, and who accepts the passer at (often literally) face value, as belonging to the same group as her- or himself. She remarks: 'As a standard feature of the passing narrative, such a triangle poses the question of the passer's "real" identity as a function of the lens through which it is viewed. Resituating the question of knowing and telling in the terms of two competing discourses of recognition, the pass emerges as a discursive encounter between two epistemological paradigms' (1994: 723–4).

The narrative scenario outlined by Robinson is rendered still more complex in the case of a man seeking to pass successfully as masculine: the threefold function she delineates may be said to be performed in fact by all men, at all times, *for it requires all three participants* – passer, dupe and member of in-group – *to both know and not-know that a masquerade of masculinity is in progress*. In this way, the man who convinces others about his masculinity may succeed also – however partially or provisionally – in convincing himself. The (male) audience for such a performance of masculinity functions as both member of the in-group (men are aware of the strategies of the performance of masculinity necessary to the individual male if he is to pass successfully as masculine) and as dupe (men accept such performance as authentic and as signifying in the performing individual an essential, inherent sense of himself as 'truly' masculine). The complexity and yet provisionality of such a scenario – especially one that must be undergone daily – imposes a continual pressure and stress on individual men that inevitably affects their psychological and physical well-being, whether in terms simply of stress-response, or in terms of feeling impelled to risky and/or dangerous practices and behaviours.

The penalties for *not* passing convincingly and successfully, however, are often immediate and unmistakable. They may range from ridicule and humiliation to physical mutilation and death (as in many cases of gay-bashing). In addition to the subjection to any physical violence, the man who is unsuccessful in passing may also suffer from the emotional and psychological effects of his failed gender strategy, leading to such further consequences as depression and possible suicide, on the one hand, and, on the other, to ever more strenuous attempts to convince both himself as well as other men that he *is*, after all, worthy of the status of masculinity. It is crucial, therefore, that one's performance of gender in order to pass persuade one's real or imaginary audience. As Schlossberg remarks: 'A convincing performance of, for example, "whiteness" or "straightness" or "womanliness" requires not just culture but skill; *the seams must not show*' (2001: 6; emphasis added).[10]

Such a performance involves more than a rhetoric of gesture and dissimulation. Speaking of gay passing for straight, Schlossberg observes: 'passing becomes a form of passive resistance, one that protects the gay subject from hostile interpretations. Passing thus can be understood at the most basic level as an attempt to control the process of signification itself. ... however, this control is often illusory or fleeting at best.' Yet, she continues, 'passing can be experienced as a source of radical pleasure or intense danger; it can function as a badge of shame or a source of pride' (2001: 3). The vertiginous combination of pleasure in passing and the constant threat of the discovery by others that this *is* simply a performance of course both underlies and characterises the superhero/ schlemiel dyad: the fear that the superhero may be revealed to be a schlemiel is countered and complemented by the pleasure of carrying out the 'deception'. Yet, as Schlossberg goes on to say:

> *Passing is not simply about erasure or denial, as it is often castigated but, rather, about the creation and establishment of an alternative set of narratives. It becomes a way of creating new stories out of unusable ones, or from personal narratives seemingly in conflict with other aspects of self-presentation. The passing subject's need to create a coherent, plausible narrative to account for his or her past suggests, on a very basic level, that every subject's history is a work in progress – a set of stories we tell ourselves in order to make sense or coherence out of a frequently confusing and complicated past. The risk and pleasure of narrative thus seems intimately connected to the risk and pleasure of passing.*
>
> *(2001: 4)*

Thus, rather than seeing the superhero as a normative masculine type, 'The Superhero' may be understood as a narrative told by the schlemiel.

In a cultural system, then, in which the discourse of gender arranges things so that the superhero male benefits to the disadvantage and detriment of the schlemiel figure, there is every reason for individual men to lay claim to the qualities of being a superhero and to distance themselves as far as possible from any potential allegation that they may in fact be schlemiels:

> *If, as we are suggesting, identity is primarily a form of storytelling, then the stakes of the story are different depending on the social location of the narrator ... the allure of rewriting identity cannot be disconnected from the very real emotional and material advantages of doing so. Obviously, the creation of a coherent narrative or stable history, a mappable trajectory, becomes all the more tempting in such cases, particularly for racialized [and homosexualised] subjects whose histories have been violently erased.*
>
> *(Schlossberg 2001: 4)*

And if constructing and publicly 'narrating' such stories derived from fear and anxiety in the individual male about being revealed as less or other than he claims to be, such that he is driven to behaviours and practices that may affect his health or even endanger his very life, he may reckon that the cost is worthwhile, given the very real benefits accruing to the superhero figure in the culture. In this way, the 'history' of the schlemiel is also tacitly erased.

Yet the schlemiel figure persists, not only as the uncomfortable other to the superhero but also as his interrogator:

> *If passing wreaks havoc with accepted systems of social recognition and cultural intelligibility, it also blurs the carefully marked lines of race, gender, and class, calling attention to the ways in which identity categories intersect, overlap, construct, and deconstruct one other [sic] ... Furthermore, the passing subject's ability to transcend or abandon his or her 'authentic' identity calls into question the very notion of authenticity itself. Passing, it seems, threatens to call attention to the performative and contingent nature of all seemingly 'natural' or 'obvious' identities.*
>
> (*Schlossberg 2001: 2*)

Historically, the figure of the schlemiel in Jewish culture has performed a similar function. Ruth R. Wisse argues that 'the impulse of the [schlemiel] joke, and of schlemiel literature in general, is to use this comical stance as a stage from which to challenge the political and philosophic status quo' (1971: 3). She remarks that the schlemiel 'is also used as the symbol of an entire people in its encounter with surrounding cultures and its opposition to their opposition' (4). She notes that in the narrative about the schlemiel, there is an irony that 'holds both the contempt of the strong for the weak and the contempt of the weak for the strong, with the latter winning the upper hand' (6). Likewise, in the discourse of gender the schlemiel figure, inferiorised and marginalised by the culture's preference, in terms of masculine ideal, for the superhero, has the potential to challenge and question, and perhaps also to interrupt, the ascendancy of the latter.

I have focused in this chapter on the superhero/schlemiel dyad because the recurrence particularly of the schlemiel in recent film[11] has been so marked, and because it is so suggestive in its implications for the structure and dynamics of the masculine. Other recent models of the masculine often convey a sense of self-awareness, frequently laced with irony; for instance, the adventure hero as exemplified by Indiana Jones (played by Harrison Ford) in three extremely popular films (1981, 1984, 1989)[12] and by Rick O'Connell (Brendan Fraser) in the two *Mummy* films (1999, 2001). That ironic self-reflexivity suggests that men in the culture have become more conscious of the performative nature of gender, and – at least in these sorts of texts – are ready to play with that notion. At the same time, contemporary performances of traditional notions of the masculine as essential and grounded in the body tend now to look nostalgic rather than convincing and affirmative.

This chapter borrows its title from Jean Renoir's 1937 film *La Grande Illusion*, in which several illusions, especially about war and its professed glories, are examined and dispelled. One of these, relevant to my theme here, is that of the overriding allegiance to class. Set during the Second World War, the film explores the ways a group of French soldiers captured by Germans establish a camaraderie that overrides their respective class origins. However, the aristocratic Captain von Rauffenstein, courteous and punctilious, assumes that his captive, the equally noble Captain de Boieldieu, shares his own upper-class attitudes, particularly his sense of being dispossessed by history and an increasing democratisation of society. Though the French nobleman acknowledges, like the German captain, the passing of his class's power and privilege, de Boieldieu's loyalties lie with his compatriots, regardless of class, rather than with his class equal von Rauffenstein, and in the end he sacrifices his own life so that two of his non-aristocratic fellow Frenchmen may escape to freedom.

The figures of the superhero and the schlemiel are foregrounded as radical and reductive representations of two ways of performing masculinity, ways that inevitably divide the men performing them into different gender classes, in a hierarchical order that privileges the superhero. The pressure that this exerts over men to strive to join the 'upper' class, as much evidence attests, has been detrimental to the health and living conditions of many men, often with consequences also for the women and children who live with them. If men's health is to improve in a general sense, the dynamic by which masculinity is produced within the discourse of gender needs to be examined and, where possible, reimagined and reformed. This does not mean that we must discard the qualities we admire in the superhero; but nor, by the same token, should we dismiss the traits of the schlemiel. Rather than draw a von Rauffenstein-like distinction between the superhero and schlemiel, characterising the former as more 'truly' masculine, we need to acknowledge that both superhero and schlemiel need and are defined by one another; and that, moreover, together both offer a wider range of behaviours, attitudes and practices to men than is generally available to males who pursue and model themselves on the superhero figure only. That is, it is not – or should not be – a question for men of being *either* the superhero *or* the schlemiel, but rather of finding a form of the masculine *that incorporates both* and makes complementary their respective individual characteristics and abilities. This would correspondingly also increase the flexibility and breadth of tolerance of men's attitudes and responses to other men, reducing the potentially destructive competitiveness inherent in patriarchal masculinity. And, in this way, we might finally allow men to develop and explore the potential of a fuller, richer and, above all, healthier masculinity.

NOTES

1 I limit instances here to the Australian context, in which I live and write; but the problem has a much wider reach, especially in Anglo cultures, with which I am most familiar.

2 See, for example, Susan Faludi's *Backlash: The Undeclared War against Women* (1992), a magisterial account of men's misgivings about women's entry into the public sphere, and their rage against it. Faludi traces a historical pattern across several cultures, focusing principally on the United States, Britain and Australia. *Backlash* should be read in conjunction with Faludi's later work, *Stiffed: The Betrayal of the Modern Man* (1999), which focuses on the USA and explores the ways that the post-Second-World-War promise of security of employment, status and lifestyle failed the generations of men whose fathers returned as soldier-heroes. In 'Backlash: Angry Men's Movements' (2004), Michael Flood examines the response of some men to the perceived ascendancy of women in such issues as family court decisions concerning the custody of children, as well as the rage engendered by the increased presence of women in the workplace.

3 See, for instance, 'Here Is the Real Masculinity Crisis', the spirited response by Brian Greig, a former Democrats Senator in the Australian Parliament, to the circulation of the idea that the crisis in masculinity is attributable to single-sex families, male children raised by lesbians, and the preponderance of female teachers in the school system.

4 See Faludi (1999).

5 It may be confirmed but not granted by women.

6 That both men and women may be represented as dismissing and humiliating the geek has its own ironies, for in an age dominated by rapidly changing technologies it seems it is the geek who shall inherit the earth.

7 Other representations in circulation often distinguish between the schlemiel proper and the *schlimazl*, one for whom luck always runs badly: 'The schlemiel

spills his wine and the schlimazl is the one he spills it on' or 'The schlemiel gets lost driving round the block, and the schlimazl is his passenger.'

8 In the past decade or so a number of films have centred on the schlemiel figure, their popularity suggesting that this representation of a problematic masculinity finds a sympathetic response in the viewing public, and especially in young males. Such films include almost all of Ben Stiller's *oeuvre*; *Napoleon Dynamite*, which gained a cult following and belongs to the subgenre of teen or college 'nerd' movies, for instance, *Superbad*; etc. Significantly, most such films close with the schlemiel gaining the privilege and appurtenances – the girl, the job, the status, etc. – of the traditional hero, suggesting an attempt both to normalise the schlemiel figure within the dynamics of masculinity and masculine power, and to bring the traditional hero and the schlemiel closer to one another in the cultural imaginary.

9 See, for example, Pope *et al.* (2002) and Fussell (1992).

10 Performing gender in order to pass is not a new concept, nor is it limited to masculinity: as long ago as 1929 Joan Rivière discussed femininity as 'masquerade' (1929). The scope of the present chapter, however, does not permit a discussion of femininity as performative. I omit, too, a consideration of the very long tradition of heteronormative masculinity as performed by gay men who seek to pass as straight, for whatever reasons – fear of homophobic violence, or of ridicule and humiliation, or a desire to preserve the status and perquisites of heterosexual masculinity, etc. – as well as the implications for the health of gay men.

11 And in television (for instance, *Everybody Loves Raymond*, 1996–2005), and in many forms of popular literature (for example, Augusten Burroughs, *Magical Thinking: True Stories* [2005]). However, considerations of space preclude a discussion of these.

12 At the time of writing, a fourth instalment, *Indiana Jones and the Kingdom of the Crystal Skull*, has just opened in Australia.

REFERENCES

Buchbinder, D. (1994) *Masculinities and Identities*. Melbourne: Melbourne University Press.

Burroughs, A. (2005) *Magical Thinking: True Stories*. New York: Picador.

Butler, J. (1993) *Bodies That Matter: On the Discursive Limits of 'Sex'*. New York and London: Routledge.

Faludi, S. (1992) *Backlash: The Undeclared War against Women*. London: Chatto & Windus.

Faludi, S. (1999) *Stiffed: The Betrayal of the Modern Man*. London: Chatto & Windus.

Flood, M. (2004) Backlash: angry men's movements. In S.E. Rossi (ed.), *The Battle and Backlash Rage On: Why Feminism Cannot Be Obsolete*. Philadelphia: Xlibris Corporation, pp. 261–342.

Foucault, M. (1979) *Discipline and Punish: The Birth of the Prison*. London: Penguin.

Fussell, S.W. (1992) *Muscle: Confessions of an Unlikely Bodybuilder*. New York: HarperCollins.

Greig, B. (2004) Here Is the real masculinity crisis. *Australian Democrats: Australian Democrats Published Articles.* Accessed 30 May 2008. http://www.democrats.org.au/articles/index.htm?article_id=18.

Kroeger, B. (2003) *Passing: When People Can't Be Who They Are.* New York: Public Affairs.

Mclean, T. (2008) Australian Blokes in Denial about Weight, 11 April. news.com.au. Accessed 30 May 2008. http://www.news.com.au/story/0,23599,23521595–36398,00.html.

New South Wales Department of Health (2001) 'Moving Forward in Men's Health'. New South Wales Department of Health. Accessed 30 May 2008. http://www.health.nsw.gov.au/health-public-affairs/men'shealth/index.html.

Pope, H.G., Phillips, K.A. & Olivardia, R. (2002) *The Adonis Complex: How to Identify, Treat and Prevent Body Obsession in Men and Boys.* New York: Free Press and Simon & Schuster.

Riley, R. (2008) Men's Health: A National Scandal, 23 March. *Herald Sun.* Accessed 30 May 2008. http://www.news.com.au/heraldsun/story/0,21985,23415571–5000112,00.html.

Rivière, J. (1929) Womanliness as masquerade. *International Journal of Psychoanalysis,* 9, 303–13.

Robinson, A. (1994) 'It takes one to know one': passing and communities of common interest'. *Critical Inquiry,* 20, 715–36.

Rosten, L. (1971) *The Joys of Yiddish: A Relaxed Lexicon of Yiddish, Hebrew and Yinglish Words Often Encountered in English, Plus Dozens That Ought To Be, with Serendipitous Excursions into Jewish Humour, Habits, Holidays, History, Religion, Ceremonies, Folklore and Cuisine; the Whole Generously Garnished with Stories, Anecdotes, Epigrams, Talmudic Quotations, Folk Sayings and Jokes – from the Days of the Bible to Those of the Beatnik.* Harmondsworth, Penguin.

Schlossberg, L. (2001) Introduction. In M.C. Sánchez & L. Schlossberg (eds), *Passing: Identity and Interpretation in Sexuality, Race, and Religion.* New York and London: New York University Press.

Ullman, S. (2001) The 'self-made man': male impersonation and the new woman. In M.C. Sánchez & L. Schlossberg (eds), *Passing: Identity and Interpretation in Sexuality, Race, and Religion.* New York and London: New York University Press.

Wisse, R.R. (1971) *The Schlemiel as Modern Hero.* Chicago and London: Chicago University Press.

FILMS AND TV PROGRAMMES CITED

La Grande Illusion, 1937, Criterion Collection.
Superman, 1978, Warner Brothers Pictures.
Superman II, 1980, Warner Brothers Pictures.
Raiders of the Lost Ark, 1981, Paramount Pictures.
Superman III, 1983, Warner Brothers Pictures.
Indiana Jones and the Temple of Doom, 1984, Paramount Pictures.
Indiana Jones and the Last Crusade, 1989, Paramount Pictures.
Everybody Loves Raymond, 1996–2005, CBS Television.
The Mummy, 1999, Universal International Pictures.

Mystery Men, 1999, United International Pictures.
Meet the Parents, 2000, Universal Pictures.
The Mummy Returns, 2001, Universal Pictures.
Zoolander, 2001, Paramount Pictures.
Spider-Man, 2002, Sony Pictures Entertainment-Columbia Pictures.
Hulk, 2003, Universal Studios.
Along Came Polly, 2004, Universal Pictures.
Meet the Fockers, 2004, Universal.
Spiderman 2, 2004, IMAX.
Napoleon Dynamite, 2004, United International Pictures.
Superman Returns, 2006, Warner Brothers Pictures.
Spider-Man 3, 2007, Sony Pictures Entertainment.
Superbad, 2007, Sony Pictures Entertainment.
Indiana Jones and the Kingdom of the Crystal Skull, 2008, Paramount Pictures.

3 MEN, PUBLIC HEALTH AND HEALTH PROMOTION: TOWARDS A CRITICALLY STRUCTURAL AND EMBODIED UNDERSTANDING

Steve Robertson and Robert Williams

INTRODUCTION

'Come on chaps, this is serious', declared a headline in *The Times* newspaper at the start of Men's Health Week 2008 in the UK (Roberts, 2008). This brief statement simultaneously homogenises men, constructs men as all being equally 'at risk' in terms of health outcomes, and suggests that men are unable, or unwilling, to look after their health and well-being – in short, it carries an implication that all men are irresponsible when it comes to self-care and promoting their own health. Such soundbites, that have reached the status of 'common-sense' and unambiguous explanations for the current 'state of men's health', rest on (and replicate) specific stereotypes of 'how men are': that is, they are built on essentialist views of masculinity that provide archetypes of men as strong, rational, stoical, aggressive, cavalier, assertive, decisive and independent, to name a few (Seymour-Smith *et al.*, 2002; Gough, 2006). These essential male characteristics often become translated in men's health rhetoric into two specific truth claims: first, men engage in activities that put them 'at risk'; second, men are reluctant to seek help for health concerns.

Conceptualising men and health in this way acts to predefine the possibilities and likely successes of attempts to improve the health of men. While this approach homogenises men as a group, it firmly places the cause of the problem within individual men's biological make-up or at least within the individual male 'psyche'. Consequently, the issues involved are already cast as 'poor behaviours' at the level of the individual and attempts at improvement are therefore aimed at facilitating individual behaviour change (indeed, health promotion literature is saturated with theoretical and empirical 'models of behaviour change'). This view of men and health is problematised by critical perspectives on health promotion/public health (to be considered shortly) that also recognise how shifts in meanings of 'health' have produced a concomitant shift in responsibility for its attainment away from government and towards the individual (or perhaps a desired shift in responsibility to the individual-required concomitant shifts in the meaning and conceptualisation of 'health').

The aim of this chapter is to consider the relationship of these critical perspectives on health promotion/public health to notions of gender and masculinities, and particularly to see what resonance these have in relation to men's own accounts. The men's accounts incorporated here are mainly from our own previous research, but we also draw on the empirical work of others. Men's accounts are utilised to generate and elucidate the discussion. In so doing, we develop arguments, briefly commenced elsewhere (Robertson, 2006a, 2007), about what critical health promotion/public health ideologies have to offer to our understanding of men and health promotion, and suggest some limitations to these. Specifically, we explore how normative conceptualisations of 'health' and 'healthy lifestyle' are endorsed and transgressed by men and the role that discourses and enactments of masculinities play in this. We then consider the importance of reinserting corporeality, male embodiment, into critical perspectives on health promotion/public health in order to refocus the 'men's health' debate on issues of social justice and social determinants without denying the importance of men's agency.

CONCEPTUALISING HEALTH

In Western societies, biomedicine is the main way that health is understood within the medical profession, by non-professional laypeople and by health researchers. The biomedical model has five principal features (Nettleton, 1995). These features, Nettleton argues, include:

1 A mind–body dualism, which suggests that the mind and body can be seen as separate entities.
2 An emphasis on mechanical metaphors, in the way the body is viewed as a machine.
3 A technological imperative, which refers to the importance of medical forms of intervention for treating the body.
4 A reductionist predisposition where there is a strong tendency within policy, research and practice to emphasise explanations on the working of body systems, which require specialist knowledge about ill health.
5 The belief in aetiology of disease which refers to the ways in which medic ine should respond to specific causes of disease.

We would suggest that this model is not a static, reified view about medical knowledge, research and practice, but these central elements of biomedicine remain. Where the medical gaze does shift away from illness, sickness, death and dying towards preventive health with social contexts, the dominant discipline for analysing the health of men, women and children within public health is epidemiology. Epidemiology is a method (and discipline) derived from medicine which involves reducing understanding human health to the quantification and recording of information regarding individuals within populations (Lupton, 2003). Not only the body and mind, but environments, localities and communities become the focus for epidemiology (Petersen, 1997). Indeed, this epidemiological information informs the development and employment of medical technologies such as screening, immunisation and, increasingly, techniques designed to eradicate 'risks' by changing the 'behaviours' or 'lifestyles' that are perceived to 'cause' illnesses within body systems.

Empirical work that explores how lay populations conceptualise health has a long history and provides an alternative, or complementary, approach to epidemiology. In reviewing this body of work, Hughner and Kleine (2004) found 18 themes that captured how health was understood. The body of empirical research on laymen's conceptualisations of health is somewhat smaller, though that which has been carried out, certainly within the 'Western world', reflects the major themes highlighted in previous work (Mullen, 1993; Saltonstall 1993; Paxton *et al.*, 1994; Sharpe & Arnold, 1999; Watson 2000; Robertson, 2006a, 2007; O'Brien, 2006; O'Brien *et al.*, 2005; Richardson, 2007). Health as 'a normal state', as the absence of illness, as the ability to function, as fitness and as 'looking good' or 'feeling good', and combinations of these, are all recurrent themes in the men's accounts found within this body of literature.

However, the way that health is conceptualised does not occur in a social or political vacuum. Numerous writers have drawn on the work of Michel Foucault in order to critically question the notion of 'health' as a stable reality that can be understood in a straightforward manner. Within Foucauldian frameworks, the way that concepts of health are understood among lay populations is not a matter of chance or a question of cultural interpretation of a 'real' physical or mental state. Rather, concepts of health, the meanings that are attached to health, are seen as historically constructed in ways that serve particular needs. In *Discipline and Punish* (1979), Foucault explores how the historical shift from sovereign power to disciplinary power required more subtle forms of control of populations, of coercion rather than explicit physical punishment. Constructing what is considered 'normal', and setting up systems of observation and examination to monitor deviance, are a key means of social control, an arm of 'governmentality', within this modern (or postmodern?) disciplinary era. Indeed, these three – normalising judgement, observation, and the examination – are seen to constitute the 'instruments of disciplinary power' (Foucault,1979: 170ff.). How health is understood, how its boundaries are defined (and redefined) and monitored, become an important site in operating this wider system of control. Armstrong (1995), in developing the notion of 'surveillance medicine', expands Foucault's work. He explores how the 'medical eye' has become cast beyond the immediate and obvious ill health of an individual towards currently 'healthy' populations. As he suggests, this historical move required a problematisation of what had previously been considered 'normal' (p. 395) and a concomitant move beyond physical signs and symptoms to an 'extracorporal space' to identify 'risk factors', linked to lifestyle choices, that 'opened up a space for future illness potential' (p. 400). It is clear from current empirical work that notions of what constitutes 'normal', and their links to lifestyle, have indeed been inculcated into men's ideas and beliefs about 'health'. For example, one man offers the following description of an idealised version of a healthy person: 'He would be just the right weight for his height. He wouldn't smoke, or drink too much. He would have regular exercise, regular amounts of sleep as well as healthy food' (Watson, 2000: 76).

In such accounts it often becomes taken as read what is meant by 'the *right* weight', 'drink *too much*', '*regular* exercise/sleep' and '*healthy* food'. These standards – as understood through recourse to Body Mass Index, units of alcohol per week, the required minutes of exercise/hours of sleep a day and familiarity with avoiding fat and eating fruit and vegetables – seem so well known as not to require further explication in such accounts (though the exact 'quantities' advised by 'official guidelines' may not always be specifically known).

Yet, recognition of these idealised health standards and norms does not reflect unquestioning compliance with them or even acceptance of them: 'I'm quite sceptical and I don't believe an awful lot of stuff they tell you. Like this type of food is good for you, then the next day it's bad for you. I'd like to think I could make up my own mind about that stuff' (Richardson, 2007: 190).

We would suggest that departure from 'healthy lifestyle' advice takes two forms: First, and fitting with Foucauldian arguments, it comes about as an act of resistance to imposed values and standards. Yet, very few examples of this are to be found in the specific research on laymen and health referenced earlier (Mullen, 1993; Saltonstall, 1993; Sharpe & Arnold, 1999; Watson, 2000; Robertson, 2006a; O'Brien, 2006; Richardson, 2007), even when specifically looked for in the data (Robertson 2007: 45). There is evidence from previous research that some men 'did not like being told what to do' in terms of lifestyle choices (Sharpe & Arnold, 1999; Gough & Conner, 2006), and this is reflected in some of our own work:

> *I just think blokes will do it when they want to do it. They won't be told. It's like anyone could tell me I need to stop smoking but I'll do it when I'm ready to stop smoking and not when someone tells me to. ... I watch all the adverts and I do think I should stop smoking. But I'm not ready to stop smoking, I might never be ready to stop. If a doctor tells me 'you need to stop smoking' then it's my decision whether I do or don't.*
>
> (Robertson, 2007: 122)

However, such accounts, as we shall see shortly, were nearly always linked to specific, pragmatic reasons for continuation of these behaviours rather than being 'resistance' for its own sake or as a political act. In recent work, barebacking (the specific and deliberate non-use of condoms during anal sex by gay men) *is* seen as being specifically used as an act of resistance to 'safe-sex' health messages and heterosexual 'norms' (Crossley, 2002). Crossley suggests that the very identification of an act as 'risky' creates the space for such resistance. Furthermore, she suggests that this is unlikely to be limited to one particular act among gay men but seems to 'be becoming more widespread amongst the population with regard to health-related behaviours such as smoking, eating and drinking' (2001: 202). In this sense, those interested in promoting the health of men, at policy as well as practice level, need to consider the generative forces behind such resistance and the ways in which these are gendered in nature.

The second departure – and we would argue more significant in terms of men's (and probably women's) health practices – emerges from the intersection of 'health' norms and values with other aspects of embodied identity. Rather than an act of resistance, empirical data suggests that non-adherence to 'healthy behaviours' is more frequently about how they are prioritised compared to alternative behaviours; in short, engagement (or not) in them is more often related to social context. As such, they should not be considered 'behaviours' in the individualistic sense but should rather be thought of as social practices established in intersubjective encounters; 'health' is not so much 'conceptualised' as 'enacted' within social contexts. Take our earlier account of a refusal to be told to stop smoking. This account was not provided in isolation, nor was it told as an act of resistance (though it did incorporate constructing a 'masculinity' based firmly in the need to show independence of thought/action). It was part of a larger narrative around smoking and health, told through two interviews with this man, which had wider context to it, as he goes on to explain:

> *Nearly every chef I know smokes because it's such a stressful job and it's just because you don't get breaks. I can do, like, 12 hours without a break, so I'll sit down for 5 minutes, have a fag and calm myself down and everything. ... It's not meant to be healthy, is it? But to me it's my form of release from the pressure of my job.*
>
> (Robertson, 2007: 50)

What we see here is not smoking as an act of resistance but smoking as an important relief from the 'stress' of work and the likely (health) impact of leaving that unchecked. In this way, health 'risks', a key concern of many Foucauldian analyses of public health (for example Lupton, 1993; Petersen & Lupton, 1996), need to be considered in respect to other potential risks, in respect to other competing discourses and men's embodied materiality. It is clear from empirical data that health is regarded, rhetorically, as a feminised concern. For example: 'Yeah, 'cause it's [health] important to women, innit, but blokes don't really bother about it. I mean speaking from my experience, like I say, I never think about it' (Robertson & Williams, 2007: 364).

Health therefore also becomes conceptualised and practised in respect to aspects of gendered identity. The construction, or presentation, of a hegemonic masculinity relies in part on a rejection of that which is feminine or feminised. Social practices, particularly for younger men, therefore often involve, even require, engagement in behaviours constructed as 'unhealthy', or 'risk-taking': 'Well, I suppose risk taking, to be seen to be one of the boys, with risky behaviour. Go out and get drunk together or, you know, take part in dangerous sports or throw yourself into the fray [fight]' (O'Brien, 2006: 73).

Yet, again, this should not always be understood as a deliberate 'performance' of masculinity. Rather, as we suggest elsewhere (Robertson, 2006a), such acts are often not consciously organised but more frequently represent what Bourdieu (1990) has termed a 'logic of practice' that develop in respect to people's social locations. As O'Brien et al. (2005: 514) suggest, what occurs, then, is a situation where health 'risks' become conceptualised (though usually unconsciously) and balanced in relation to a 'hierarchy of threats' to masculinity.

MORALITY AND 'GOOD CITIZENSHIP'

In Foucauldian analysis, the ultimate regulation of populations within public health and health promotion policies and practice comes not simply from external surveillance but from the way established notions, norms and standards related to such external surveillance become accepted by individuals and the degree to which self-surveillance is then achieved (Petersen & Lupton, 1996). Lifestyle risk discourses carry with them moral connotations and messages about the appropriate and required (health) behaviours expected of 'good citizens' (Lupton, 1993). These are found in men's empirical accounts in terms of what people 'ought to do', what they know they 'should' do, or indeed in terms of presenting themselves as virtuous citizens who do 'the right thing', or do not do the 'wrong' thing:

> *When you've had a few [drinks], responsibility goes out the window and it's not until the morning you say* 'I shouldn't have *had the last couple'.*
> *I know cigarettes are bad for me, people die from smoking* ... I might know the answer *but doing it, like* ...
> *I'm in a position where I'm concentrating more on my health,* watch certain things *in relation to food. I've* given up *smoking a long time ago and hopefully will* cut down *on drinking* ...
> *(Richardson, 2007: 188, 189, 177)*

However, as highlighted towards the end of the previous section, these normative discourses about what constitutes a 'good citizen', in terms of healthy lifestyle 'behaviours', can clash with the social practices required within hegemonic masculine discourses; an issue that has received very little attention to date by writers taking a Foucauldian approach to public health/health promotion.

We have suggested elsewhere that this creates a dilemma for men. On one hand, as real (hegemonic) men, they cannot be seen to be too concerned about 'health' (feminine) issues but, on the other hand, as 'good citizens', there is a moral obligation to show concern and engage in 'healthy' practices. We have termed this the 'don't care/should care' dichotomy (Robertson, 2006a, 2007; Robertson & Williams, 2007). Within this previous analysis, we have also recognised the importance of a further dichotomy within health promotion developed in the work of Robert Crawford (1984, 2000). He suggests that within contemporary capitalism there is a requirement on individuals to be both producers (workers) and consumers. This requires 'two fundamentally different behavioural patterns' (2000: 221): first, behaviours that sustain a disciplined workforce – the standard 'healthy lifestyle behaviours' identified earlier; second, behaviours that feed consumption – 'loosening the restraints of utility, rationality, and self-denial and activating tastes for pleasure, variety and convenience'.

This creates a discursive imperative in terms of health (and other social) practices towards the need for both 'control' and 'release' by individuals in the pursuit of good, moral, citizenship:

> *It's like the smoking, I told you about that. I gave up when the second one [baby] was born ... I thought I have got to be serious about this and I stopped ... eventually. I still like to go on the lash [drinking alcohol] on a Saturday night. You've got to, really, I mean you have got to have a good time some time, but not all the time. In moderation, if you know what I mean.*
>
> *(Robertson & Williams, 2007: 364)*

In Crawford's analysis, rather than seeing non-compliance to 'lifestyle' advice *only* as a form of resistance, both compliance and non-compliance with health promotion standards and messages are recognised as system requirements for sustaining contemporary capitalism. Indeed, as others have suggested (Eakin *et al.*, 1996: 163), what occurs is a situation where 'transgression' ('release') therefore becomes simultaneously health-damaging yet health-enhancing in terms of the feeling of well-being and emancipation it provides:

> *I eat healthy food generally and I cheat now and again. Alcohol's bad for you, but we all drink, mostly everyone I know likes a drink, 'cause it's good for you, it actually cheers you up. We've got like this throwaway society and I think people's perceptions are changing, everybody wants everything yesterday. People want to gain as much as possible materialistically, physically and emotionally. And that's it, get fit one day, get drunk the next, buy the best house in the country the day after you know, and that's a full life.*
>
> *(Robertson, 2007: 46)*

What is important here is how these narrative accounts of 'morality' and 'good citizenship' are sustained and rejected through recourse to discourses of appropriate gendered social practices as alluded to earlier. Particular circumstances require more 'control' than 'release' and facilitate compliance with standard 'healthy lifestyle' advice. For example, a group of male firefighters in one study were

> *unique in having a supportive peer group who shared an interest in health matters and were similarly motivated to preserve health and their work identity ... consulting even for trivial problems, or to prevent health problems, was important in allowing them to maintain their health and thus retain their job.*
>
> *(O'Brien et al., 2005: 514, 515)*

These men can resist discourses of health as a 'feminised' issue by recourse to a (more powerful) gendered discourse of men as responsible professionals in a job that generates significant social (and reasonable economic) capital. Other situations, where some 'risks' are measured against others, lead to practices that specifically transgress 'healthy' lifestyle standards. As one man highlights when he recounts his experience in the army:

> You're in a group of 30 people and they are all trying to be the macho man, the Alpha male. And you don't want to go against the grain cause then you're automatically picked on. So you're, 'Go on, I'll have that cigarette, and I'll have that one extra beer' ... If you're not in the streamlined group, you're shunned, you just don't fit. And if you don't fit then ...
>
> (Robertson, 2007: 51)

It is this socially contingent nature of health practices, and its relationship to 'doing gender', that enables men to engage in contradictory 'behaviours' in varying circumstances. Hegemonic masculine discourses, and rejection of these, are alternatively (and sometimes simultaneously) used to support compliance with, and to support transgression from, 'healthy behaviours'. Indeed, it may not be uncommon to find the same firefighters engaged in some of the 'macho' practices present in the Army narrative on a night out in order to avoid similar sanctions and maintain 'status' with their peers[1] (see also Gough & Edwards, 1998).

For us, a further advantage of Crawford's model over a Foucauldian analysis lies in the implicit judgements made about compliance/resistance. In the Foucauldian framework, compliance to health promotion advice seems to carry with it an implication that one is 'giving in' to normalising discourses and are therefore in some sense a 'conscript', or worse still, a willing participant, in disciplining processes; in short, compliance means that you are, either by design or desire, part of the 'problem' of systems of governance. Conversely, and again by implication, transgression is represented as the wise choice for those intelligent enough to resist dominant discourses and thereby challenge state control of and intervention in their lives. Crawford, on the other hand, while acknowledging the problems inherent in extending 'health' to cover ever increasing areas of life, prompts recognition that both compliance with 'healthy' standards *and* transgression from (resistance to) these are requirements of contemporary capitalism; that is to say, no judgements

(implicit or otherwise) are made about individual acts of compliance or resistance. Rather, the main concern is that individuals,
and specific social groups, are made morally responsible – and to
feel responsible – for health inequities that are actually socially/
politically produced and originate from the pursuit of contemporary capitalism.

In terms of the health of men, this can be seen to be at play
in the way that men's reduced longevity (compared to women)
is often constructed as being directly related to their 'risk-taking' behaviour, reluctance to adhere to advice and unwillingness
to seek help (for example, Peate, 2004; Davis, 2007). Very little work to date on men's health promotion identifies the significance of socially structured factors as determinants of men's
health practices/outcomes and therefore seeks social/political
rather than individually based interventions.

THE PLACE OF 'BODIES'

One of the greatest contributions of Crawford's work has been to
elucidate the meanings attached to health and health promotion
as social practice and to critically examine the relationship of the
discourses that surround these to the current neo-liberal political climate. Yet, we would suggest that Crawford's model also has
limitations. In constructing health *only* as a linguistic/discursive
practice (Crawford, 2006: 405), there is a neglect of the material, corporeal elements that are also significant in generating
health outcomes and that need consideration in promoting the
health of men. It is not *only* the health discourses of 'discipline
and pleasure' that are entangled to create a central contradic-
tion in contemporary social order (Crawford, 1999: 364). We
agree that traditional positivist, and naïve realist emphasis, on
the body within biomedicine is unhelpful in helping us understand the links between the structural, the social and the body.
However, the materiality of physical bodies is important, as is
the embodiment of gender, in understanding men's health experiences. Indeed, it is often these material elements, these corporeal, physical bodies, which are affected within the inequitable
social arrangements generated and fostered through neo-liberal politics. We are not alone in suggesting this as a limitation
of Crawford's work. In debate around these points between

Crawford (1999) and Williams (1998; 1999b), the latter high-lights how 'A critical theory of health ... must go beyond this focus on issues of *discourse, meaning, valuation and metaphor*, to the material body which underpins, yet extends far beyond and is never entirely encompassed by, these socio-cultural and histori-cal constructions' (p. 368).

There is similar dominance given to linguistic/discursive practices in Foucauldian writing where the body, literally, never 'materialises': 'If the body can only be known through a descrip-tive language (the "gaze" for the last two centuries) then it is futile to speculate on "essential features" that could never be described' (Armstrong, 1997: 21).

This is a big 'if', and the materiality of the body cannot be dis-pensed with so easily just because our descriptive language and symbolic understanding of it vary over time. We would argue that while the *reductionist* (*naïve*) realism within biomedicine is limit-ing, a *critical* realist framework can actively assist our understand-ing of bodies, and health, as both representational and material (Robertson, 2006b; Williams, 1999a, 2002). Within such a frame-work, there is recognition of a 'real' physical body, and underlying corporeal processes, yet also that our knowledge and understand-ing of these is always subject to change. In critical realist terms, the 'real' body, and its processes, reside in the realm of the intran-sitive (what is), whereas our knowing about these always remains in the realm of the transitive (what we understand about what is) (Sayer, 2000: 10). Thus, as the meaning and language we attach to bodies changes historically it does not mean that bodies and their corporeal processes themselves change. This is not a slide back into biomedically-based reductionist approaches – the dis-courses, meanings and symbolic representations relating to health and bodies are crucial – but it is a move away from extreme con-structionist approaches that fail to deal adequately (if at all) with issues of physicality and materiality. It is also important to recog-nise that the representational and the material aspects of bodies are not readily separable; that is, in practice, they are integrally entwined. Given that what we know about the 'real', material, body exists in the realm of the transitive, our understanding of it is inevitably wrapped up in discourses and representations. Yet, this should not lead us to abandon attempts to obtain a 'practi-cally adequate' (rather than definitively 'true') understanding about these material elements (Sayer, 2000: 40ff.).

This framework has more resonance with men's accounts of their lived experience; with their own embodiment. As shown with the firefighters above, men display concern with corporeal processes that are recognised as important in sustaining daily (pragmatic) embodiment, and this becomes increasingly significant if people begin to show the effects of bodily fragmentation:

> *Originally, I had a weak [sore] ankle for about 14 months and kept going regularly to see Dr S. After 14 months I said to him, 'I'm getting sick of this now. I'm coming every month, having this injection, doing this and that. I've strapped up me boots, I'm even getting smaller boots to keep me ankle tight and solid, what are we gonna do about it?' So he says, 'Well, we'd better do a biopsy'. So they put me in touch with someone else, did the biopsy and it was cancer.*
>
> (Robertson, 2006b: 439)

Similar accounts can be found in the majority of empirical work on laymen's conceptualisations of health. In these accounts, as Williams (1999a: 373) suggests, the body has 'a will and indeed a voice of its own'. The meaning this man attached to his discomfort (and the meaning the doctor attached to it) did not alter the underlying corporeal processes; indeed, discourse and language were not required at all *a priori* to give voice to the weakness/discomfort. In this sense, the body should also be recognised as an entity subject to its own governance (Turner, 1984).

While a little less immediate in nature, the anticipation of bodily fragmentation is also not *only* a discursive fabrication developed as a form of governance mediated through discourses of 'health'. What we might currently call 'genetic predisposition' to development of particular types of bodily fragmentation has a basis in underlying corporeal processes, no matter what language and meaning we attribute to them and how this might change over time (it may be understood as something other than 'genetic predisposition' in the future). A degree of surveillance and self-surveillance in such circumstances should not therefore *only* be interpreted as 'social control' or as *only* bowing to the system requirements of contemporary capitalism. Rather, it can be interpreted, at least in part, as a logical act to promote self-survival: 'It [his willingness to engage in health screening] goes back to the experience of the heart [attack] with my father, like, so I wasn't willing to take the chance ... I mean we all want to live as long as we can and be as healthy as we can' (Richardson, 2007: 230).

There has been recognition in previous writing on surveillance medicine, and associated processes of medicalisation, that men's bodies have been notable by their absence (Rosenfeld & Faircloth, 2006: 1). The reasons for this are undoubtedly complex. One suggestion is that Foucauldian work has failed to intersect with more recent sociological focus on the embodiment of everyday life (Rosenfeld & Faircloth, 2006: 2) and our discussion here concurs with this view. We also see another process at work directly relating to the role of gender in this process of concealing male bodies. As we have outlined elsewhere, the embedding of gendered hierarchies within health structures creates a particular slant to the 'medical gaze' (Robertson, 2007: 135). Under patriarchy, it is a (hegemonic) male gaze that undertakes observation and examination and a (hegemonic) male 'norm' by which others (women, non-hegemonic men) are measured[2] (White, 2002: 131). In this way, as those wielding the tools and being at the top of a gendered 'hierarchy', it is less likely that (hegemonic) men themselves would become the subject of such instruments of disciplinary power. As one man comments: 'But perhaps men won't go, they need ... if it's voluntary to go and have your men's health check then perhaps a high proportion of men won't go ... If they did regular health checks then the response rate wouldn't be high, they don't want to change, men' (Robertson, 2007: 129).

Such concealment of (some) men from health surveillance services and processes can then represent a double-edged sword. The structural embedding of concealing male bodies helps maintain the hegemonic (male) privilege to continue one's life with minimum interference. Yet it also creates the potential for early detrimental changes to corporeal processes, and their subsequent longer-term outcomes, to go unrecognised.

The argument here is *not* that 'well-man checks', surveillance and screening programmes are a panacea for promoting the health of men (or women and children) – indeed, we have been strong critics of such approaches elsewhere (Williams & Robertson, 2006; Robertson & Williams, 2007; Williams & Robertson, forthcoming; see also Gough, 2006). Rather, the argument is that these approaches should not *simply* be understood as an element of governmentality or *only* as an impossible attempt to resolve the contradictory problems associated with contemporary capitalism and its concomitant requirement for balancing 'healthy' control and release. What we are suggesting is that such approaches should not be ruled out *per se* as having no value, or even as being 'health-damaging'. The bigger issue here is about whether surveillance and screening programmes represent the most effective ways of significantly improving the health of men (and others), under which circumstances and for which men, and whether there are more effective approaches that could be taken, such as the reduction of poverty.

In line with this approach, we suggest that there should be a shift in emphasis from 'lifestyle' to 'life-chances' in the way that 'men's health promotion/public health' is conceptualised and practised. This shift would facilitate a primary emphasis on men's lived environment, on issues relating to housing, education and transport, on the impact of racism, homophobia and class difference. It would require consideration of how the structural embedding of gendered hierarchies within a neo-liberal political system influences the opportunities and choices ('chances') available to individual and specific groups of men in respect to their health practices and outcomes. Yet it also retains a focus on how individual men might wish to respond to corporeal threats, or actual bodily changes and fragmentation. It allows for consideration of how individual experience and history might influence health practices and outcomes through compounding, or facilitating resistance to, the impact of structural factors; it does not rule out the role that men, as active agents, have (and wish to have) in taking/creating chances to determine their health practices and outcomes – though it would not construct these as matters of 'free choice'. In short, it allows exploration of both structure and agency, and their relations, in respect to men and health.

CONCLUSION

Foucauldian perspectives on public health/health promotion have provided crucial insights into how discursive conceptualisations of normative 'healthy lifestyles' can be deployed (in part) as a means of controlling population groups. Yet, the overemphasis on non-compliance as (and only as) resistance, and an implicit judgement that resistance to such discourses is the politically correct choice, seems to provide only partial insight into the complexities involved in understanding men's health practices. In addition, little work within this Foucauldian framework has considered, or looked to explore, how discourses around 'healthy lifestyles' coalesce and/or clash with gendered, masculinity discourses, in which social contexts, and with what outcomes.

Crawford's (1984, 1999, 2000, 2006) work allows us to see how both compliance with, and transgression from, normative health promotion guidelines are necessary to fulfil the system requirements of neo-liberal, contemporary capitalism. This removes implicit judgements about compliance and non-compliance to such guidelines while maintaining a focus (found also in Foucauldian perspectives) on how moral responsibility for health is shifted away from governments and on to individuals. This approach has more resonance with men's own accounts, where the interplay of 'control' and 'release' can be found. These accounts also show a two-way relationship where narratives of 'control' and 'release' are supported by recourse to discursively normative gendered (hegemonic male) practices, and vice versa.

The difficulty remains, however, that both these perspectives rely only on the discursive meanings attached to 'health'. In doing so they fail to recognise the importance of corporeality, materiality and men's embodied selves. While certainly not wishing to collapse back into reductionist biomedical perspectives, we would wish to retain an emphasis on men's accounts of their lived, bodily experiences. We suggest critical realist frameworks allow us to consider the importance of both discursive constructs and physicality in relation to men and their health. These frameworks can be deployed in the practice of men's health promotion by focusing away from individualist notions of 'lifestyle' (and its associations with 'choice') towards a more structural emphasis on 'life-chances'. Doing this facilitates the appropriate consideration of issues of structure and agency, and their interrelations, with regard to men's health practices and outcomes.

NOTES

1 We would suggest that it is this contingent nature of social practice that explains why measuring attitudes/beliefs as predictors of health behaviours has such limited utility.

2   This can still be the case when the individual health professional involved is
    female, as power is still being exerted to serve patriarchal purposes (Davis,
    1995).

REFERENCES

Armstrong, D. (1995) The rise of surveillance medicine. *Sociology of Health &
    Illness*, 17(3): 393–404.
Armstrong, D. (1997) Foucault and the sociology of health and illness: a prismatic
    reading. In A. Petersen and R. Bunton, *Foucault: Health & Medicine*. London:
    Routledge, pp. 15–30.
Bourdieu, P. (1990) *The Logic of Practice*. Cambridge: Polity.
Crawford, R. (1984) A cultural account of health: control, release and the social
    body. In J.B. McKinlay (ed.), *Issues in the Political Economy of Health Care*.
    London: Tavistock, pp. 60–103.
Crawford, R. (1999) Trangression for what? A response to Simon Williams. *Health*,
    3(4): 355–66.
Crawford, R. (2000) The ritual of health promotion. In S.J. Williams, J. Gabe & M.
    Calnan (eds), *Health, Medicine and Society: Key Theories, Future Agendas*. London:
    Routledge, pp. 225–35.
Crawford, R. (2006) Health as meaningful social practice. *Health*, 10(4): 401–20.
Crossley, M.L. (2001) 'Resistance' and health promotion. *Health Education Journal*,
    60(3): 197–204.
Crossley, M.L. (2002) The perils of health promotion and the 'barebacking' back-
    lash. *Health*, 6(1): 47–68.
Davis, C. (2007) Men behaving badly. *Nursing Standard*, 21(21): 18–20.
Davis, K. (1995) *Reshaping the Female Body: The Dilemma of Cosmetic Surgery*.
    New York: Routledge.
Eakin, J. Robertson, A., Poland, B., Coburn, D. & Edwards, R. (1996) Towards a criti-
    cal social science perspective on health promotion research. *Health Promotion
    International*, 11(2): 157–65.
Foucault, M. (1979) *Discipline and Punish: The Birth of the Prison*. Harmondsworth:
    Peregrine.
Gough, B. (2006) 'Try to be healthy, but don't forgo your masculinity': decon-
    structing men's health discourse in the media. *Social Science & Medicine*, 63:
    2476–88.
Gough, B. & Conner, M.T. (2006) Barriers to healthy eating among men: a qualita-
    tive analysis, *Social Science & Medicine*, 62(1): 387–95.
Gough, B. & Edwards, G. (1998) The beer talking: four lads, a carry out and the
    reproduction of masculinities. *Sociological Review*, 46(3): 409–35.
Hughner, R.S. & Kleine, S.S. (2004) Views of health in the lay sector: a compilation
    and review of how individuals think about health. *Health*, 8(4): 395–422.
Lupton, D. (1993) Risk as moral danger: the social and political functions of
    risk discourse in public health. *International Journal of Health Services*, 23(3):
    425–35.
Lupton, D. (2003) *Medicine as Culture: Illness, Disease and the Body in Western
    Societies* (2nd edn). London: Sage.

Mullen, K. (1993) A Healthy Balance: Glaswegian Men Talking About Health, Tobacco and Alcohol. Aldershot: Avebury.

Nettleton, S. (1995) The Sociology of Health and Illness. Cambridge: Polity.

O'Brien, R. (2006) 'Men's Health and Illness: The Relationship Between Masculinities and Health'. PhD thesis, Social & Public Health Sciences Unit, University of Glasgow.

O'Brien, R., Hunt, K. & Hart, G. (2005) 'It's caveman stuff, but that is to a certain extent how guys still operate': men's accounts of masculinity and help seeking. Social Science & Medicine, 61(3): 503–16.

Paxton, S.J., Sculthorpe, A. & Gibbons, K. (1994) Concepts of health in Australian men: a qualitative study. Health Education Journal, 53(4): 430–8.

Peate, I. (2004) Men's attitudes towards health and the implications for nursing care. British Journal of Nursing, 13(9): 540–5.

Petersen, A. (1997) Risk, governance and the new public health. In A. Peterson & R. Bunton (eds), Foucault: Health and Medicine. London: Routledge, pp. 189–206.

Petersen, A. & Lupton, D. (1996) The New Public Health: Health and Self in the Age of Risk. London: Sage.

Richardson, N. (2007) 'Men's Health Practices and the Construction of Masculinities'. PhD thesis, Faculty of Health & Social Care, University of the West of England.

Roberts, Y. (2008) 'Come on chaps, this is serious'. The Times, 7 June.

Robertson, S. (2006a) 'Not living life in too much of an excess': lay men understanding health and well-being. Health, 10(2): 175–89.

Robertson, S. (2006b) 'I've been like a coiled spring this last week': embodied masculinity and health. Sociology of Health & Illness, 28(4): 433–56.

Robertson, S. (2007) Understanding Men and Health: Masculinities, Identity and Well-being. Buckingham: Open University Press.

Robertson, S. & Williams, R. (2007) Masculinities, men and public health policy. International Journal of Interdisciplinary Social Sciences, 2(2): 361–8.

Rosenfeld, D. & Faircloth, C.A. (2006) Medicalised masculinities: the missing link. In Rosenfeld & Faircloth (eds), Medicalised Masculinities. Philadelphia: Temple University Press.

Saltonstall, R. (1993) Healthy bodies, social bodies: men's and women's concepts and practices of health in everyday life. Social Science & Medicine, 36(1): 7–14.

Sayer, A. (2000) Realism and Social Science. London: Sage.

Seymour-Smith, S., Wetherell, M. & Phoenix, A. (2002) 'My wife ordered me to come!': a discursive analysis of doctors' and nurses' accounts of men's use of general practitioners. Journal of Health Psychology, 7(3), pp. 253–68.

Sharpe, S. & Arnold, S. (1999) Men, Lifestyle and Health: A Study of Health Beliefs and Practices. London: Social Science Research Unit, University of London.

Turner, B.S. (1984) The Body and Society: Explorations in Social Theory. Oxford: Blackwell.

Watson, J. (2000) Male Bodies: Health, Culture and Identity. Buckingham: Open University Press.

White, K. (2002) An Introduction to the Sociology of Health and Illness. London: Sage.

Williams, S.J. (1998) Health as moral performance: ritual, transgression and taboo. *Health*, 2(4): 435–57.

Williams, S.J. (1999a) Is anybody there? Critical realism, chronic illness and the disability debate. *Sociology of Health & Illness*, 21(6): 797–819.

Williams, S.J. (1999b) Transgression for what? A reply to Robert Crawford. *Health*, 3(4): 355–66.

Williams, S.J. (2002) Corporeal reflections on the biological: reductionism, constructionism and beyond. In G. Bendelow, M. Carpenter, C. Vautier & S. Williams (eds), *Gender, Health and Healing*. London: Routledge.

Williams, R. & Robertson, S. (2006) Masculinities, men and promoting health through primary care. *Primary Health Care*, 16(8): 25–8.

Williams, R. & Robertson, S. (forthcoming) Masculinities, 'men's health' and policy: the contradictions in public health in the UK. *Critical Public Health*.

4 BUGGING THE CONE OF SILENCE WITH MEN'S HEALTH INTERVIEWS

John L. Oliffe

INTRODUCTION

The interview is one of the most powerful qualitative methods which takes us into the world of the participant and allows us to see the content and patterns of their experience(s) (McCracken, 1988). Moreover, interviews offer access to participants' ideas, thoughts and memories in their own words (Reinharz, 1992) and are an excellent medium with which to discover the subjective meanings and interpretations that participants give to their health and illness experiences (Denzin, 1989). That said, challenges routinely emerge in and around men's health interviews. Indeed, in writing the earlier drafts of this chapter, I grappled with the enormous complexity about what is – or at least to my mind, should be – a relatively simple and straightforward enterprise: talking with, and listening to men. To search for a starting point and chapter plan I took the liberty of a somewhat self-indulgent mid-afternoon nap to dream up what I could reasonably say, and how that information might be made accessible to novice and expert interviewers, as well as those who locate themselves along that continuum. My first thought was somewhat tangential and took the form of Maxwell Smart, a character spawned in the 1960s television sitcom *Get Smart*. Throughout my primary-school years Max (aka Agent 86) was a constant in my life. I wouldn't say that I was particularly fond of Max – or the show, for that matter – instead, his presence was predetermined for most of the pauper television generations who grew up without colour on their screens, let alone the programme choice (and the repetition) later afforded by cable. My after-school intrigue for *Get Smart* centred on the *cone of silence*, arguably Max's favourite gadget, which was designed

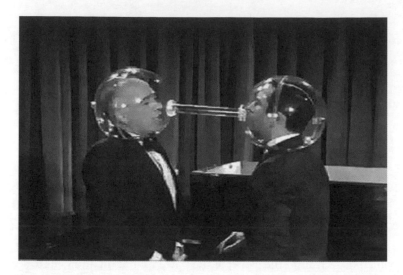

Figure 4.1   The cone of silence

Source: (http://alistair.cockburn.us/images/Maxwell_Smart_in_a_cone_of_silence.jpg)

to allow him and the chief of spy operations to talk privately. Of course, the reruns confirm the cone of silence as faulty and an inefficient means of communication, yet Max never lost faith in it. There were many versions, and Figure 4.1 depicts one of the more sophisticated models. The cone of silence running gag involved a third character showing up to echo the two speakers' conversation.

The cone-based interactions embody many of the challenges that occur when men are asked to talk about their health. The struggles of muted, muffled and filtered conversations, incongruence between messaging and reception, the need for a third party to translate what is *really* said, and the primacy of confidentiality when men reveal ordinarily secret information permeate many research interviews. However, I want to suggest that qualitative researchers have great potential and an obligation to be at the forefront of clearing some of those muddy waters and disrupting dominant discourses that espouse real men as stoic and alexithymic[1] by collecting and making available first-hand accounts of what men say, as well as what they don't say. In other words, I am advocating that researchers become more skilful in *bugging the cone of silence*. To detail how we might best advance this endeavour I have interspersed some of my experiences related to interviewing men in three vignettes, along with an overview of what has already been said in the literature. In doing so I have triaged two macro issues to locate the subsequent discussion that focuses on being there as a researcher in the interview. Rather than any grandiose illusions about providing definitive answers, I share what follows in the hope of ensuring continued discussion of these and related issues well beyond the pages of this chapter.

MACRO ISSUES: ENTERING INTERVIEW WORLD

Many issues emerge around talking with men about health. First and foremost, the researcher generally initiates that dialogue, and as the person asking men to speak about their health the interviewer is accountable for much more than merely asking questions. I have included two inextricably linked issues – *writing yourself in* and *participant recruitment and gatekeepers* – to detail some considerations about the researcher's roles and responsibilities around men's health interviews.

Writing yourself in

Aside from introducing this chapter in the first few paragraphs I took the opportunity, at least briefly, to *write myself in* to what follows. This is appropriate, and some would argue obligatory, if one subscribes to the point of view that researchers and participants engage with a synchronous process of data production to co-create knowledge about men's health and illness experiences (Abu-Lughod, 1993; Manderson *et al.*, 2006). Some degree of author self-disclosure affords the reader insights to *who* collected and analysed the data and ideally makes available not just *what* the researcher knows, but *how* they know it (Reinharz, 1992). Unfortunately, most empirical journals don't have the space for such detail, and even if they did, the minutiae would be inherently messy in multi-author publications, where the findings are influenced and produced by a team of writers rather than one person. Routinely, reflexivity is the term used by researchers to signal their all-encompassing ontological and epistemological qualitative savvy, but the specific details are positioned as considerations, best residing in the pages of methods-based articles. Even in qualitative theses and dissertations that afford author

details to the examiners (and other readers), the empirical findings lay in wait, the *meat* separate from the methods chapter(s)
where the intricate details of data collection and analyses feature. This is not a criticism per se, but rather an observation that
readers are rarely afforded information about who conducts the
interviews and analyses, and these details, or lack thereof, can
imply that objective, uniform or common-sense interpretations
are derived from what men say about their health practices.

Congruent with Finlay and Gough's (2003) assertions about
the limits of reflexivity, I am not advocating radical reflexivity
that places the researcher's experiences rather than the participants' under investigation, at centre stage. Nor am I suggesting
a prevailing, privileged self-awareness and promotion by and for
the researcher (Davies, 1999). However, the predominance of
white, middle-class, educated men currently doing masculinities
and men's health research needs to be acknowledged as influencing both the theoretical conceptualisations and empirical products derived from *their* gendered analyses. I am not arguing for
or against researcher diversity here, but instead want to suggest
renewed commitment to context because the interviewer's markers (i.e., sexuality, culture, gender, class-based ideals) demand
attention throughout the entire research process as they can
shape all the interactions that occur. For example, leading up to,
as well as during data collection, long before the writing up of
the study findings and their dissemination as articles, chapters
and books, there are inevitably questions about who is conducting the interview. The researcher's end-product to chronicle their
participation in the study, *writing yourself in*, which I am promoting here, is therefore intertwined with the entire project, including the entry point of most studies, *participant recruitment and
gatekeepers*. As Robertson (2006) has previously demonstrated,
researchers should not only accept, but also describe how their
gender performances and relations around and within the formal
interviews strongly influence men's health studies.

Participant recruitment and gatekeepers

The challenges of recruiting men for interview-based research has
been linked to dominant ideals of masculinity, including men's
resistance to women partners' coercion strategies (Brown, 2001),

long work hours and limited flexibility in scheduling *extra* activities (Butera, 2006), refusal to accept potential surveillance by others (Adler & Adler, 2001) and concerns about knowledge deficits in discussing specific health topics (Laws & Drummond, 2002; Oliffe & Mróz, 2005). Men's outright refusal to participate in interviews has also been interpreted as doing masculinity – signifying independence, rationality and control in saying *no* (Butera, 2006). The aforementioned factors link recruitment challenges to men's masculine identities within specific studies. However, it is important to acknowledge that significant others', as well as dominant discourses about masculinity, influence men's health practices and their related talk (see Gough, 2006, 2007; Robertson, 2007). In qualitative interview studies, researchers disrupt many of the masculine ideals they propose to investigate by suggesting men should talk about their health. Third-party endorsement and permission can be central to securing men's buy-in to this atypical and perhaps suspect activity (Gibson & Denner, 2000; Butera, 2006). Therefore, researchers' relationships with gatekeepers, who by definition are individuals that have the power to grant or deny access to people for the purposes of research (Minichiello, 1990), often influence the involvement of potential participants and ultimately determine the feasibility of completing interview studies (Adler & Adler, 2001; Yong, 2001; Oliffe, 2003; Oliffe & Mróz, 2005; Butera, 2006). A field-work example is shared in Vignette 1, *Whose men are they?*,

---

Vignette I   Whose men are they?

I first learned about the power of gatekeepers when recruiting men from prostate cancer support groups (PCSGs) for my doctoral work. My attempts to access participants were closely monitored by a group secretary who incessantly quizzed me about my background and motives for conducting a study that involved talking with men. During the six months of attending group meetings, routinely and relentlessly, he quipped about the unusualness of an emergency room *male* nurse being interested in, let alone wanting to talk to men, about their prostate cancer. He openly joked with the other men at the group about me living in a trendy

Vignette I   (*continued*)

affluent suburb (implicitly 'othering' me by contrasting my assumed middle class with the predominance of working-class attendees and the lower socio-economic status of the suburb wh ere the meetings took place). His innuendo and line of questioning continued, until finally he initiated a private conversation during which he asked me, 'Do you have a girlfriend?' My affirming 'yes' was followed by his subtle demand for assurances that neither the group's efficacy nor his facilitation style were the true focus of my study. Aside from the secretary's obvious suspicion, his tactics for expressing his doubts ensured my outsider, subordinate status at the group. I continued to attend the meetings until eventually he agreed to *give* me an opportunity to explain my study and invite attendees to participate. He labelled and introduced that agenda item as 'John Oliffe's Mystery Talk', further piquing the mystique of an outsider. As I began a much rehearsed monologue an unexpected gatekeeper – a woman employee of the Anti-Cancer Council of Victoria and a guest speaker for that particular PCSG meeting – emerged with lightning speed and an accusatory tone to intercept the third word of my second sentence with the question, 'Do you have permission from the Anti-Cancer Council of Victoria to access *our* group?' A sinking feeling overtook me and an uncontrollable staccato infiltrated my voice as I attempted to repair the fractured sentence explaining that I had university ethics approval and the formal permission of the group secretary to talk with the men about my study. Clearly rattled, and with my research life flashing before my eyes, I stammered through the remainder of my invitation to the potential study participants before meekly taking my place at the back of the room. The silence grew until the secretary stood before the men and eloquently suggested that it was not his perception, nor was it mandated that the Anti-Cancer Council of Victoria had ownership of the group. The approving nods of the men rallied to support the secretary, as my unlikely new-found ally looked in my direction and further asserted, 'She can't stop the men from talking with you if they want to'. His pseudo-endorsement of my study pre-empted the enrolment of five men that very day, a windfall return in qualitative terms.

to illustrate how gatekeepers can emerge and operate, to be complicit in sustaining dominant masculine ideals. These issues extend to other scenarios, including men's partners and physicians who also often act as gatekeepers, either endorsing particular projects and encouraging men to participate, or inversely, questioning the need for their men to be directly involved.

At one level, the secretary's need to know, jibe and test me could be interpreted as well-meaning strategies to protect the interests of the group and the men attending the meetings from any unethical research. Masculinities were clearly at play here, and as Schwalbe and Wolkomir suggest, signifying masculinity routinely occurs when men research men, and a prevailing gender order requires that men must 'signify possession of an essentially gendered self that makes our placement in a particular category right and proper' (2001: 90). Although I attempted to fit within the group, it was a woman espousing authority over the men's collective that afforded me the leverage to be less subordinate in the gender order that operated at the group. It was also evident that both gatekeepers were protective of their men, keen to avoid any interview-induced emotion that might manifest as residual melancholy, sadness and/or anger for the men who talked with me. Similarly, prostate cancer physicians routinely enrol their patients in randomised control trials, but tend to dismiss and deny access to qualitative researchers. Again, masculine hierarchies operate here to privilege science and affirm interview-based research as soft and subordinate. Implicit to many gatekeepers' protective actions are affirmations that men don't talk, and concern that those who do may be derailed by such unhealthy introspection.

Similar gatekeeper interactions have been reported by women researchers who conducted interview studies with men. For example, in a study of Australian based rural farmers, Pini (2005) described how men routinely signalled their heterosexual identity in front of fellow males to assert their machismo, and positioned themselves as busy, powerful, knowledgeable, important, and expert through various tactics to further reinforce their status as men. Vivian Yong (2001) described a lack of gatekeeper understanding, unequal power relations and bureaucratic resistance when attempting to recruit survivors from PCSGs for her doctoral study. I expect that the specific expressions and experiences vary depending on gatekeeper–researcher gender dynamics, and in the case of Yong (2001), her Chinese ethnicity may have also influenced the PCSG fieldwork. Although formal gender comparisons would no doubt reveal intriguing differences, two themes prevail that offer important considerations for both men and women researchers. First, interactions with gatekeepers yield important data and insights about the impact of gender, and it should be expected that some traditional gender roles and relations will reign to downplay and perhaps balance the disruption that researchers cause by soliciting men's talk (Pini, 2005). Rather than contesting power differentials, being complicit and appealing to men's sense of prestige and power to gain their interest in participating (both directly with individuals and through gatekeepers who are willing to assert their own powerful influence on men) can yield significant dividends (Butera, 2006). Although the inverse has also been argued – that appealing to hegemonic masculinities can be counter-productive since it is often associated with health-averse practices (Gough, 2006) – potential solutions may be muted by assumptions that masculine ideals always potentiate and advance men's pathologies rather than their health (Oliffe et al., 2008; Oliffe, Gerbrandt et al., forthcoming; Oliffe, Ogrodniczuk et al., forthcoming). Second, researcher presence and subtle persistence demonstrates commitment to the population being studied. This is an important consideration because gatekeepers are typically invested in their men and/or a greater cause (e.g., prostate cancer screening, access to health-care services, smoking cessation) and studies that have the potential to directly benefit participants and/or raise public awareness about men's health issues can mobilise strong grass-roots support. Developing and sustaining these relationships can also be integral to disseminating the study findings to communities and soliciting the involvement of stakeholders in activating understandings as interventions. In summary, it is clear that around men's interviews, there is much to interpret about gender relations and the co-construction and negotiation of masculinities.

MICRO ISSUES: INSIDE THE INTERVIEW

Talking about self-health is an unusual experience for most men, especially when the conversation is devoid of therapeutic recommendations and outside the familiar zone of fact-finding and problem-solving (Brown, 2001; Oliffe & Mróz, 2005). Typically, biomedical science and positivist thinking predominate in men's talk about taking up health-care services and self-disclosure to professionals in the hope of finding a remedy. Men's relationships to research and what counts as knowledge also tend to focus on the causes and cures of disease rather than their illness experiences. Embodied here are masculine ideals about how to interpret, act on and talk about health and illness. For example, men's dialogue is typically problem-based and constructed around existing pathologies rather than illness prevention. This was illustrated in a comparison of middle-aged healthy men and men who had experienced a myocardial infarction (MI), which revealed MI as the linchpin for participants discussing their health (Brown, 2001). Men's objective talk is also routinely demanded by health service providers in clinical settings through direct questioning focused on narrowing down the cause of specific ailments. The inverse applies in qualitative interviews because the questions and answers are not linked to producing a diagnosis or prescribing therapy, and the data gathered are disseminated as patterns and themes rather than a means to objectively measure relationships and test hypotheses. As such, the processes and products of qualitative interviews are at odds with most men's health talk and perceptions of worthwhile scientific research.

Ideally, ongoing informed consent can satisfactorily locate qualitative interviews for men who participate. However, men often agree to be interviewed because they are paid for their time, told that it will be good for them and/or because they want to tell their story to raise awareness and help or teach others (Kimmel, 1994; Oliffe & Mróz, 2005). Regardless of why men agree to participate, the onus is on the interviewer to normalise and promote men's talk within what is often the foreign terrain of qualitative interviews. Many factors influence participant disclosures, some of which are discussed in the following two sections, *location(s)* and *identity markers, conversations, questions and photographs*.

Location(s)

The physical location in which the interview takes place affects the dynamics of the interview, and influences participant–researcher power relations (Sin, 2003). The use of the interviewer's workplace privileges the interviewer, while a coffee shop or park provides a more neutral public space that can affect confidentiality and potentially inhibit dialogue about private and emotive topics (Manderson *et al.*, 2006). Men may also experience reduced agency as a by-product of being interviewed in a public place (Lee, 1997). The use of an interviewee's home can bring the interviewer into the participant's private life, revealing the class and social status of the interviewee through the type of housing, as well as clues to masculine identity and history through the personal artefacts that are routinely open to comment (Manderson *et al.*, 2006). Ideally, participants are afforded their choice of location for the interview; however, securing safe places can take precedence for researchers in some circumstances. For example, unwelcome advances and mis-interpretations of interviews as *dates* were detailed by Lee (1997) in a study of workplace sexual harassment for which she interviewed men. The qualitative methodology underpinning the study design also influences the researcher's preference for where interviews take place. Vignette 2, *The interviewer as visible minority*, is drawn from an ethnographic study of senior South Asian Canadian immigrant men to demonstrate how location can also encompass culture and social class to influence participant–researcher power relations and the interview data (Oliffe *et al.*, 2007).

Vignette 2 illustrates how power relations invariably influence what men reveal. Ironically, I perceived myself as powerless and perpetually awkward in trying to guess how best to demonstrate respect and embody SA cultural sensitivities at the temple. Yet the interviewee positioned me as superior, and did not want to waylay me with what he assumed I would interpret to be uneducated and uninformed opinion. In addition, data from the second interview (conducted by the SA woman) revealed other factors which likely influenced the participant in our earlier interview. Specifically, the man explained that he had inherited his healing skills from an old and dying man in SA, the therapeutic powers of which were disarmed if he received payment for his services. Therefore, my interview may have been interpreted as a form of surveillance or stealing in which the man's knowledge was being assessed against and/or potentially claimed by Western medicine. In addition, accepting the $20 honorarium for that interview may have contra-vened the conditions under which his healing powers were inher-ited and subsequently operated. Throughout the study, SA cultures predominated, and the norms that abided hierarchies routinely governed what was shared by the men. My experiences in conduct-ing the SA men's study consistently illustrated the complexities of

Vignette 2   The interviewer as visible minority

Participants for a South Asian Canadian immigrant men's study were recruited from health clinics that operated at Sikh temples. Sikh temples (see Figure 4.2) are scattered throughout Canada and afford opportunities for worship, social and community connection, and the sharing of traditional South Asian (SA) rituals and meals.

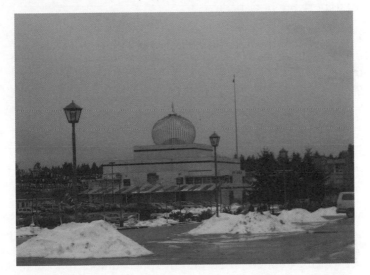

Figure 4.2   A Sikh temple in Canada

As had become routine, I arrived at the clinic to see a roomful of people having blood pressure and blood sugar checks, and my Punjabi/English-speaking SA colleagues (a man and a woman) excitedly reported that lots of men had volunteered to be interviewed. A well-known traditional SA healer who provided remedies for a multitude of minor ailments was among the volunteers, and he agreed to talk with me through an interpreter. The SA male interpreter, the participant and I adjourned to a small room adjacent to the clinic to conduct the interview. The discussion began well, and matter-of-factly I asked about the man's experiences with SA traditional medicines and natural remedies. To my surprise, he denied any

Vignette 2   (continued)

knowledge of such things and continued to do so, despite numerous rephrasings of the question and explicit assurances that I was keenly interested to hear about his perspectives. Eventually, the participant politely closed the interview, summating, 'I am an uneducated man and you are a doctor ... the Canadian health care system is great and I am very grateful to be living in Canada'.

Distracted and a little confused by what had happened, I had lunch at the temple's communal hall *(Langar)* with my two SA colleagues as the interviewee re-emerged to offer me tea, smiling as he filled my cup. My SA colleagues assured me that the man had not lied per se, but rather, as a mark of respect recognised that he had nothing legitimate to offer me. They also reaffirmed the appropriateness of my wearing a tie at the temple, suggesting it was expected by the SA men to whom I wanted to talk. My SA female colleague, perhaps sensing my helplessness, re-interviewed the same man, one-on-one, and produced another narrative in which numerous traditional SA remedies intertwined with details about the participant's health practices were highlighted.

power which extended far beyond the physical location where the interview was conducted.

Similarly, in a study assessing Italo-Australian men's access to prostate cancer information, Laws and Drummond (2002) described how culture- and gender-informed region-specific differences in the extent to which men expressed a willingness to self-disclose. Men from rural Italy, aligned to a traditional masculinity, displayed a restricted indulgence in personal matters, particularly those related to health. Although researcher–participant ethnic matching might offer a solution, Chih Hoong Sin, a male researcher of Chinese ethnicity, commented otherwise after interviewing an elderly Chinese man, suggesting, 'The assumption was that I would understand things that would not need to be articulated' (2003: 310). When researching men from different ethnic backgrounds, it is important to examine diversity within as well as between cultures. These examples illustrate how participant–researcher locations are relative and contextual, and strongly implicated in the much debated interviewer inheritance question, *Who gets what in men's health interviews?* Gender is also central to thīs debate. For example, same-sex interviews with men have been employed as a means of building rapport, and women interviewers are also a popular choice because men are espoused as more open to talking with women about personal issues (Williams & Heikes, 1993). Women are also depicted as empathetic listeners who facilitate men's discussions, and in doing so perpetuate stereotypical gendered roles (Winchester, 1996), whereas men may be more comfortable discussing feminine topics, including family life (Broom *et al.*, 2007). Men participants can also exhibit social desirability bias, quickly gauging what sits well with the interviewer and performing accordingly particularly when interviewed about gender-sensitive topics by female interviewers (Broom *et al.*, 2007; Schwalbe & Wolkomir, 2001; Williams & Heikes, 1993). There is some evidence that joint mixed-sex interviews can reveal less stereotyped gender behaviours among men than individual interviews, regardless of the sex of the interviewer (Seale *et al.*, 2008). Interviewer age and social class can also impact what is shared in men's interviews. For example, in an Australian study examining the experiences of adults living with impaired mobility, younger interviewers lacked a colloquial style and did not engage in self-disclosure when compared with older and more experienced interviewers (Manderson *et al.*, 2006).

In sum, Vignette 2, along with an emergent literature, confirms that the influence of location exists beyond the physical to include the participant–researcher intermix of culture, class and gender, all of which significantly influence *what* men say about health as well as *how* they say it.

Identity markers, conversations, questions and photographs

Qualitative men's health interviews demand a unique form of dialogue, and some observations and interviewer strategies for promoting participant's talk are shared in the literature. These include recommendations to pay close attention to identity markers which men use in interviews to let the researcher know who they are, as well as to locate and justify their testimony (Broom *et al.*, 2007).

There is great value in listening to men talk on their own terms about what is important to them, because invariably, sexuality, achievements, assets and other key masculine indicators are signalled in participant narratives. Subtle self-disclosures can affirm the participant's identity as multi-faceted and contingent on much more than health status or the focus of the study for which he is being interviewed (Oliffe & Mróz, 2005; Schwalbe & Wolkomir, 2001). Often, identity markers are inadvertently interpreted by researchers as *dross* (data that do not explicitly relate to the research questions) and instinctively interviewers are tempted to guide the interviewee back, or towards the topic under investigation. However, important details are embedded in these cues and auto-narratives, many of which can be formally analysed to further reveal connections between masculinities and men's health practices. The interviewer is also read by the participant. Therefore, providing assurances from the outset that there are no wrong answers or views, and demonstrating active listening by tailoring comments and questions based on what markers are disclosed (as opposed to asking 'one size fits all' generic questions), can explicitly privilege the interviewee as an expert, key informant.

Feminist researchers suggest that conversations rather than questions best avoid the participant becoming a passive member of unequal status (Oakley, 1981). Conversations provide a sense of connectedness facilitated through free interaction between the researcher and participant (De Laine, 1997). Reinharz labels this 'interviewee-guided investigation', noting that it encourages participants' experiences and the audibility of multiple voices in a person's speech to be central to the interview (1992: 21). Feminist researchers have long known the value of in-depth interviews which promote the sharing of stories and information (Oakley, 1981; McKee & O'Brien, 1983; Cunningham-Burley, 1984). That said, there are a number of important considerations regarding conversations in men's health interviews. One benefit of conversations is that they dislocate many men's previous health talk within traditional medical consultations whereby the *patient* describes symptoms or problems and avoids disclosing emotional or experiential perspectives. Social constructionist researchers are epistemologically driven to facilitate conversations that explicitly avoid questions and answers. In terms of expectations Cameron (1998) suggests that conversations are normative for some men (and women), while Kvale (1996) espouses survey questionnaires as the most appropriate means to bypass men's linear talk in capturing their perspectives. The best way forward, at least from my perspective, is to anticipate men's conversations as contextual and potentially different from those of women, particularly when the predetermined topic relates to self-health. Characteristics of men's talk including dynamism language and turn-taking styles of exchange may also be used by men to anchor their testimony. These linguistic styles can afford familiar masculine territory, assuring men that their talk is not feminine even though the topic of health typically is. I suspect that most men's health researchers would consider a good interview to be one where the participant rather than the researcher takes up the majority of the talk time. Inversely, researchers routinely accept that there is much to be learned when men's comments and responses are brief. Although some characteristics of men's talk might not fit with feminine ideals about what constitutes conversation, they often embody common forms of masculine talk.

Whilst not wanting to suggest the need for a tonic or remedy to increase or change men's talk, a number of techniques can assist greatly in securing productive interviews. Strategies for asking interview questions include invoking what other men have said in previous interviews to aid men in divulging personal and emotional information (Schwalbe & Wolkomir, 2001; Hutchinson *et al.*, 2002). Commentaries and hypotheses regarding other men's health practices can also yield important *shadow* data to reveal participants' perceptions about what constitutes masculine ideals, as well as their relationships to those characteristics and discourses. The use of mirroring – or integrating the participant's gendered patterns of speech to the language of the interview – can also be an effective means to build rapport with the interviewee (Butera, 2006). Prompts, probes and loops are useful strategies. Prompt questions such as, 'How did that happen?' or 'When did that occur?' encourage participants to describe and detail their experiences. Probes such as 'What is an example of that?' or 'Why do you think that happened?' can be used to encourage reflection and introspection about particular issues and events. Probes can also be used to move men back and forth between past, present and future to reveal changes over time in their perspectives about health and illness (Hutchinson *et al.*, 2002; Oliffe, Bottorff *et al.*, 2008). When particular questions are avoided or misinterpreted by participants, loops can be used to rephrase questions and circle back to a topic of interest.

Aside from strategies for asking interview questions, engaging other methods, including photographs, may further facilitate men's talk (Schwalbe & Wolkomir, 2001). Photo-elicitation, also referred to as photo interviewing (Hurworth, 2003) and photo-feedback (Sampson-Cordle, 2001), is based on the simple idea of inserting photographs into research interviews (Harper, 2002). Participant-produced and professionally produced photographs have been used in qualitative men's health studies addressing prostate cancer (Oliffe, 2003; Oliffe & Bottorff, 2007; Oliffe, 2009a, b) and smoking among new fathers (Johnson, Oliffe *et al.*, forthcoming). Vignette 3, *Smokin'*, is drawn from a study investigating men's

---

Vignette 3   Smokin'

A 27-year-old new father took a series of photographs with a disposable camera after he was asked to contribute images to an exhibition entitled 'Smoking through the Eyes of Fathers'. The man worked as a carpet cleaner and shared details about his workspaces. Figure 4.3 showed the dashboard of his work van, and the participant(P)–researcher(R) dialogue that followed the insertion of the image in the interview is included below.

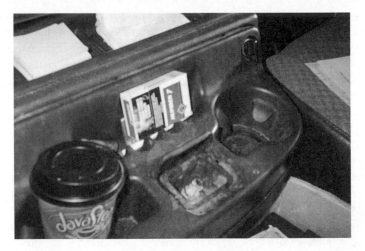

Figure 4.3   Dashboard of new father's work van

P: That one is a picture of one of the trucks that I drive at work ... and it's like all of them – I drive all of them but that's just one particular one with my coffee, my smokes and I literally got a cigarette, figured this whole picture thing is about cigarettes so I figured I would just take a picture of the pack and the ashtray.

R: So you would switch vehicles – like, you don't have the same vehicle all the time at work?

P: No ... I float.

R: OK, um, so I was just wondering about – so do you always have the coffee with a cigarette?

P: Oh yeah, first thing in the morning.

R: OK, and what's it like if you don't have the coffee or you don't have a cigarette?

P: I feel very irritable [laughs].

R: OK, and if you had to choose between one of the two, which one would you take?

P: For the most part I would take the smoke, 'cause coffee is not really a big heartthrob to me, I can just drink it or not drink it, it's nice to have but if I don't have it I'd go and have it ... they [coffee and cigarettes] just seem to go together just like beer and smoking goes together.

R: And is this, um, when you're in your more usual smoking spaces?

P: Yep, pretty much, 'cause I can't really smoke while on the job 'cause I'm cleaning other people's carpets so can't really do that.

R: Is there ever anyone else with you in the van?

P: Not usually, um, hardly ever really, it's just mainly one guy per van but sometimes they do throw people into two-man crews and that's what they're actually doing with me every Friday so ... I'm in a two-man crew with a guy that just quit smoking so he doesn't actually mind me smoking beside him 'cause he still sits there, chews his gum, has his patch on, doesn't faze him.

R: OK, so it doesn't affect your smoking

P: Not really.

R: And did you ask him first?

P: No I didn't have to actually, 'cause he was joking around about it before I even decided to get into the van and he was like, 'no smoking' and I was like, OK, so I sat there, I got out actually while we were waiting for one of our jobs and I got out of the van and he's like, oh, 'I was just joking, you can come back in', so ... I didn't want to stand outside so I sat back in the van.

R: OK, so you would have accommodated him if he asked?

Vignette 3   (continued)

P: Oh, yeah.

R: And why is it important to you?

P: Well, it's just courtesy, it's something people should be doing every day, just like if I asked someone not to smoke around my baby, I'd hope that they'd be that courteous to me and – it's what one person would do, do unto you, type thing, do unto another.

---

tobacco use during their partner's pregnancy and postpartum, in which photo-elicitation methods were used to connect masculinity and men's smoking behaviours (Oliffe, Bottorff *et al.*, 2008; Oliffe, Bottorff *et al.*, forthcoming).

The narrative was unpacked incrementally, and initially the cigarettes and ashtray were depicted as obvious – speaking for themselves – but the details emerged about the intricacies of the participant's job and his relationship with a co-worker who had recently quit smoking. Embedded here are the rules of engagement, including the specificities of courtesy and fair play between a smoker and a quitter. In closing, the participant hoped the same courtesies would be afforded to his child by others. The potential deleterious effects of smoking and second-hand smoke on both men seem lost here. However, dominant discourses about fathering emerge in the participant's commitment to protecting his newborn from other people's smoke. Vignette 3 illustrates how the participant's work, fathering ideals and health practices are invoked by the photograph, and despite some closed-ended interview questions and brief responses, a great deal of information is provided about how the stigma around smoking can be internalised, negotiated and downplayed by compartmentalising it as an activity operating outside dominant discourses about fathering.

In summary, diverse strategies should be used to foster and facilitate men's talk, and the interview content and processes (both verbal and non verbal) should be recognised as gendered performances in and of themselves.

CONCLUSION

In closing, I want to briefly address some empirical, methodological and theoretical considerations in *bugging the cone of silence* on men's health and illness talk. First, empirically, more attention should be paid to listening intently and tapping into all the resources that are embedded in men's narratives. Although valuable insights have been highlighted about men's health-related experiences, there is a strong imperative to design and implement viable gender-sensitive interventions and services that meaningfully engage specific groups of men. I suggest this, at least in part, because funded health research increasingly demands much more than thick descriptions about the problems with men's self-health. As Smith *et al.* (2008) suggest, by drawing on the accounts of men, many of whom are self-directed problem solvers and consumers of health care, important lay answers can be identified in men's narratives. Said another way, if men's health interviews focus entirely on problems, then qualitative research will forever be at the periphery pointing, rather than contributing, to solutions to advance the well-being of men. Second, methodologically men's health interviews have relied heavily on both the researcher and participant being in the same physical locale to talk in real time. If we expect men to talk but recognise that many won't participate in face-to-face qualitative interviews, strategies are needed to overcome the inherent limitations of talking potentially with outliers. Whilst acknowledging that being there in the interview yields wonderful insights and contextual understandings, there are more time-efficient and cost-effective virtual means to retrieve and analyse existing – as well as solicit new – data. Facilities such as Skype™ offer a means to audibly and visually connect with and interview men from all over the world. Blogs can provide a repository of text data that is easily retrieved in addition to affording opportunities to access men and communities that might not be available for face-to-face interviews. One advantage of virtual mediums is anonymity, and this alone can free some men to discuss ordinarily private health matters. New entry points such as these might enable researchers to recruit distinctly different groups of men to better understand diverse phenomena in various locales. Third, theoretically, masculinities frameworks (Connell, 1995) have provided a robust platform to more deeply consider men's narratives. However, there is a pressing need to talk with boys and men of different generations, geographies, social classes and cultures to inductively derive understandings about what constitutes dominant ideals of masculinity, and the implications of these ideals for how men experience and express health and illness. Therefore, the interviewee's masculine ideals should be better understood in describing the plurality across men's lives and the differences and patterns that prevail within and between men.

In conclusion, the danger of not taking up these and other challenges is that researchers may inadvertently subscribe to, and perhaps perpetuate, a static means and end for men's qualitative health interviews. Clearly, there is a need to *get smart* in recognising and mobilising what happens both in and around the *cone of silence* from which men's health talk routinely emerges.

NOTE

1 Normative male alexithymia is described as a non-pathological state in which men are unemotional and non-expressive. This phenomenon is thought to impact on the quality of men's lives and their social networks, and can be quantified through a validated instrument (Levant 2006).

REFERENCES

Abu-Lughod, L. (1993) *Writing Women's Worlds: Bedouin Stories*. Berkeley: University of California Press.

Adler, P.A. & Adler, P. (2001) The reluctant respondent. In J.F. Gubrium & J.A. Holstein (eds), *Handbook of Interview Research: Context and Method*. Thousand Oaks, CA: Sage, pp. 515–36.

Broom, A., Hand, K. & Tovey, P. (2007) The role of gender, environment and individual biography in shaping qualitative interview data. *International Journal of Social Research Methodology*, 1–6. http://dx.doi.org/10.1080/13645570701606028, accessed 7 April 2008.

Brown, S. (2001) What makes men talk about health? *Journal of Gender Studies*. 10(2): 187–95.

Butera, K. J. (2006) Manhunt: the challenge of enticing men to participate in a study on friendship. *Qualitative Inquiry*, 12(6): 1262–82.

Cameron, D. (1998) Gender, language, and discourse: a review essay. *Signs*, 23(4): 945–73.

Connell, R. (1995) *Masculinities*. Oxford, England: Polity.

Cunningham-Burley, S. (1984) 'We don't talk about it': issues of gender and method in the portrayal of grand-fatherhood. *Sociology*, 18(3): 325–38.

Davies, C. (1999) *Reflexive Ethnography: A Guide to Researching Selves and Others.* London: Routledge.

De Laine, M. (1997) *Ethnography Theory and Applications in Health Research.* Sydney: MacLennan & Petty.

Denzin, N. (1989) *The Research Act: A Theoretical Introduction to Sociological Methods* (3rd edn). Englewood Cliffs, NJ: Prentice Hall.

Finlay, L. & Gough, B. (2003) *Reflexivity: A Practical Guide for Researchers in Health and Social Sciences.* Oxford: Blackwell Science.

Gibson, M. & Denner, B. J. (2000) *Men's Health Report 2000: The MAN Model – Pathways to Men's Health.* Daylesford, Australia: Centre for Advancement of Men's Health.

Gough, B. (2006) 'Try to be healthy but don't forgo your masculinity': deconstructing men's health discourse in the media. *Social Science & Medicine*, 63(9): 2476–88.

Gough, B. (2007) 'Real men don't diet': an analysis of contemporary newspaper representations of men, food and health. *Social Science & Medicine*, 64(2): 326–37.

Harper, D. (2002) Talking about pictures: a case for photo elicitation. *Visual Studies*, 17(1): 13–26.

Hurworth, R. (2003) Photo-interviewing for research. *Social Research Update* (University of Surrey), 40: 1–4.

Hutchinson, S., Marsiglio, W. & Cohan, M. (2002) Interviewing young men about sex and procreation: methodological issues. *Qualitative Health Research*, 12(1): 42–60.

Johnson, J.L., Oliffe, J.L., Kelly, M.T., Bottorff, J.L. & Le Beau, K.T. (forthcoming) The readings of smoking fathers: a semiotics analyses of tobacco cessation images. *Health Communication.*

Kimmel, M. (1994) Masculinities as homophobia: fear, shame, and silence in the construction of gender identity. In H. Brod & M. Kaufman (eds), *Theorizing Masculinities.* Thousand Oaks, CA: Sage, pp. 119–41.

Kvale, S. (1996) *Interviews: An Introduction to Qualitative Research Interviewing.* Thousand Oaks, CA: Sage.

Laws, T.A. & Drummond, M. (2002) The complexities of interviewing Italo-Australian men about sensitive health issues. *Contemporary Nurse*, 12(2): 144–54.

Lee, D. (1997) Interviewing men: vulnerabilities and dilemmas. *Women's Studies International Forum*, 20(4): 553–64.

Levant, R.F., Good, G.E., Cook, S.W., O'Neil, J.M., Smalley, K.B., Owen, K. & Richmond, K. (2006) The normative male alexithymia scale: measurement of a gender-linked syndrome. *Psychology of Men and Masculinity*, 7(4): 212–24.

Manderson, L., Bennett, E. & Andajani-Sutjahjo, S. (2006) The social dynamics of the interview: age, class, and gender. *Qualitative Health Research*, 16(10): 1317–34.

McCracken, G. (1988) *The Long Interview.* Newbury Park, CA: Sage.

McKee, L. & O'Brien, M. (1983) Interviewing men: 'taking gender seriously'. In E. Gamarnikov, D. Morgan, J. Purvis & D. Taylorson (eds), *The Public and Private.* London: Routledge.

Minichiello, V. (1990) *In-depth Interviewing: Researching People.* Melbourne: Longman.

Oakley, A. (1981) Interviewing women. In H. Roberts (ed.), *Doing Feminist Research.* London: Routledge & Kegan Paul, pp. 30–61.

Oliffe, J.L. (2003) 'Prostate Cancer: Anglo-Australian Heterosexual Perspectives.' Doctoral dissertation, Deakin University; Geelong, Victoria, Australia.

Oliffe, J.L. (2009a) Health behaviors, prostate cancer and masculinities: a life course perspective. Men and Masculinities, 11(3): 346–66.

Oliffe, J.L. (2009b) Positioning prostate cancer as the problematic third testicle. In A. Broom & P. Tovey (eds), Men's Health: Body, Identity and Social Context. London: John Wiley, pp. 33–62.

Oliffe, J.L. & Bottorff, J.L. (2007) Further than the eye can see? Photo elicitation and research with men. Qualitative Health Research, 17(6): 850–8.

Oliffe J.L., Bottorff, J.L., Kelly, M. & Halpin, M. (2008) Fatherhood, smoking and pho-tovoice: an approach to analysing participant produced photographs. Research in Nursing and Health, 31, 529–39.

Oliffe, J.L., Bottorff, J.L., Johnson, J.L., Kelly, M., LeBeau, K. (forthcoming). Finding smoking spaces in British Columbia: The perspectives of new fathers. Qualita-tive Health Research.

Oliffe, J.L., Gerbrandt, J., Bottorff, J.L & Hislop, T.G. (forthcoming) Health promo-tion and illness demotion at prostate cancer support groups. Health Promotion Practice.

Oliffe, J.L., Grewal, S., Bottorff, J.L., Luke, H. & Toor, H. (2007) Elderly South Asian Canadian immigrant men: confirming and disrupting dominant discourses about masculinity and men's health. Family and Community Health, 30(3): 224–36.

Oliffe, J.L., Halpin, M., Bottorff, J.L., Hislop, T.G., McKenzie, M. & Mróz, L. (2008) How prostate cancer support groups do and do not survive: a British Colum-bian perspective. American Journal of Men's Health, 2(2): 143–55.

Oliffe, J. & Mróz, L. (2005) Men interviewing men about health and illness: ten lessons learned. Journal of Men's Health & Gender, 2(2): 257–60.

Oliffe, J.L., Ogrodniczuk, J., Bottorff, J.L., Hislop, T.G. & Halpin, M. (forthcoming) Connecting humor, health and masculinities at prostate cancer support groups. Psycho-Oncology.

Pini, B. (2005) Interviewing men: gender and the collection and interpretation of qualitative data. Journal of Sociology, 41(2): 201–16.

Reinharz, S. (1992) Feminist Methods in Social Research. New York: Oxford University Press.

Robertson, S. (2006) Masculinity and reflexivity in health research with men. Auto/ Biography, 14(1): 1–18.

Robertson, S. (2007) Understanding Men and Health. Masculinities, Identity and Well-being. Maidenhead: Open University Press.

Sampson-Cordle, A. V. (2001) 'Exploring the Relationship between a Small Rural School in Northeast Georgia and its Community: An Image-based Study using Participant-produced Photographs.' Doctoral dissertation, University of Athens; GA, USA.

Schwalbe, M. & Wolkomir, M. (2001) The masculine self as problem and resource in interview studies of men. Men and Masculinities, 4(1): 90–103.

Seale, C., Charteris-Black, J., Dumelow, C., Locock, L. & Ziebland, S. (2008) The effect of joint interviewing on the performance of gender. Field Methods, 20(2): 107–28.

Sin, C.H. (2003) Interviewing in 'place': the socio-spatial construction of interview data. Area, 35(3): 305–12.

Smith, J.A., Braunack-Mayer, A., Wittert, G. & Warin, M. (2008) 'It's sort of like being a detective': understanding how Australian men self-monitor their health prior to seeking help. *BMC Health Services Research*, 8(56). Advance online publication, doi 10.1186/1472-6963-8-56, accessed 23 May.

Williams, C.L. & Heikes, E.J. (1993) The importance of researcher's gender in the in-depth interview: evidence from two case studies of male nurses. *Gender & Society*, 7(2): 280–91.

Winchester, H.P.M. (1996) Ethical issues in interviewing as a research method in human geography. *Australian Geographer*, 2(1): 117–31.

Yong, V.T. (2001) Interviewing men on sensitive issues. *Contemporary Nurse*, 11(1): 18–27.

Part 2

POPULAR CONCEPTIONS OF MEN'S HEALTH AND WELL-BEING

5 MEN'S NEGOTIATIONS OF A 'LEGITIMATE' SELF-HELP GROUP IDENTITY

Sarah Seymour-Smith

INTRODUCTION

The focus of this chapter is on men's participation in self-help groups and how this identity is potentially problematic for men. This focus is relevant in the light of claims that aspects of hegemonic masculinity inhibit men from self-care and healthy lifestyles (Gough, 2006). Men's involvement in self-help groups potentially challenges the view that 'real men' don't engage in health-care practices.

Since the late 1990s we have witnessed a significant increase in the number of support and self-help groups (Gray & Fitch, 2001), and researchers have suggested that such groups are becoming increasingly popular (Bui *et al.*, 2002). Most research suggests that cancer patients' involvement in self-help groups results in improved quality of life and greater compliance with therapy, and there is even some indication that attendance may improve survival (Anderson, 1992; Fitch, 2000). However, despite this general increase in attendance, certain members of society are believed to be less willing to attend support groups than others. One strand of research has investigated the reasons people give for joining, or not joining, a self-help group. Barriers to participation include gender, ethnicity, socio-economic factors, a perception of adequate support at home, and non-attendance owing to the severity of the illness (Bui *et al.*, 2002). Significant to this chapter was the observation that men participate in self-help groups and support groups to a lesser extent than women (Thiel de Bocanegra, 1992). For instance, women outnumber men at a ratio of four to one in their attendance of cancer support groups (Cella & Yellen, 1993). Yet, little is known about the reasons why these documented differences in men and women's levels of attendance at self-help groups exist.

My aim in this chapter is to explore men and women's presentation of their self-help group identities. However, owing to the restrictions of space, women's accounts are often referred to rather than presenting this data corpus in any detail. This is important for a number of reasons. First, little empirical evidence is offered to support claims that researchers make about gender differences in self-help group attendance. Theoretical suggestions have included the proposal that women prefer to focus on needs rather than on the more rational, action-orientated activities said to appeal more to men (Gray *et al.*, 1997; Adamsen *et al.*, 2001). A further line of investigation suggests that men's reluctance to attend self-help groups is linked to issues of autonomy and self-reliance. For example, Adamsen *et al.* consider the 'prevailing social norm that delimits gender positions, with society finding it more socially acceptable for women rather than men to speak about and react to illness' (2001: 529).

Second, the distinctions between self-help groups and support groups are often blurred in the literature. Each group generally consists of a number of individuals who are in the same position, such as those suffering from the same disease or aiming to overcome a certain problem. The major difference is that support groups are facilitated by professionals and are linked to a social agency or formal organisation, whereas self-help groups are not (Gray & Fitch, 2001). The issue of definition is important because a key focus of research undertaken on support groups has concerned the format of the meetings. For example, some programmes have specifically attempted to attract men in a 'gender-sensitive' way. For example, a Danish intervention designed a group programme that included physical training and lecture sessions (Adamsen *et al.*, 2001). Their findings suggest that this type of action-oriented programme appealed more to male cancer patients. Adamsen *et al.* (2001) suggested that this might reflect different styles of male and female coping. Other research also draws upon this hypothesis, viewing men as thriving on problem-focused coping strategies and interventions that stress regaining control and action-orientation (Vingerhoots & Heck, 1990). The familiar suggestion is that men prefer to take action whereas women tend to place more value in sharing and talking through personal experiences (Klemm *et al.*, 1999). However, research on members of self-help groups is sparse (Gray & Fitch, 2001). Furthermore, there has been little detailed consideration of the ways in which men's self-help group identities are linked to masculinity (Gray *et al.*, 2002).

A third limitation with the existing research is that few studies have explored comparatively how men and women experience support/self-help groups. What tends to happen is that claims are made about gender without any grounding in empirical evidence. Thus future research needs to incorporate a relational element to better explain gendered differences.

Against this backdrop, my focus on men and women's presentation of their self-help group identities allowed me to progress the research in a number of ways. Using discursive psychology (Edwards & Potter, 1992) to conduct a fine-grained analysis of interviews with a small sample of men who belonged to a testicular cancer self-help group and women who belonged to a breast cancer self-help group allowed me to place more emphasis on the performance of participants' self-help group identities. In addition, neither of the groups that I worked with were led by a professional body, affording participants the freedom to negotiate their self-help group identity as they chose, and my analysis focuses on this issue. Furthermore, the inclusion of women allowed me to compare gendered accounts in order to provide insight into what was specific about masculinity (Frosh *et al.*, 2002). Following Connell (1987), masculinity is conceptualised as both personal and social and produced in relation to structure and power. This chapter draws upon the work of Wetherell and Edley (1998), who have developed Connell's explanation of hegemonic masculinity to gain more insight into how masculinities emerge in practice, and situates this work within the context of men's health.

THE STUDY

The data for this study consisted of tape-recorded interviews conducted with four men (aged between 26 and 31) who belonged to the same testicular cancer self-help group and seven women (aged 33 to 64) who belonged to the same breast cancer self-help group. While women are included as a point of reference, it is men's accounts which are prioritised here owing to space restrictions. Both groups were situated in the Midlands area of the UK. All the participants were white. 'Cal' is the leader of the testicular cancer group. Some of the men refer to him in their accounts.

The researcher (white and female) was aged 36 at the time of the interviews. Ethical approval from the relevant university ethics committee was gained and all participants consented to taking part in the study. Confidentiality was assured and anonymity provided through the use of pseudonyms. Each interview lasted between 50 minutes and two hours. The tapes were transcribed using a simplified version of the scheme developed by Gail Jefferson (Potter, 1996).

The interview schedule was divided into sets of questions which initially focused on the participants' illness story. Towards the end of the interview I asked specific questions about involvement in self-help groups. The analysis then focuses on both specific, researcher-led, interview questions about participants' involvement in self-help groups and participants' own orientations to this topic which occur throughout the interview.

I explore men and women's self-help group identities through the close analysis of discourse. Discursive psychology (Edwards & Potter, 1992) provides a systematic framework for the analysis of interactional data. The specific analytic approach adopted in this chapter synthesises fine-grain conversation analysis/ ethnomethodology with an interest in wider cultural, historical and power relations (see Wetherell, 1998 for a detailed defence of this synthetic view). Such an approach enables me to combine an interest in the wider discourse of men's health with the situated, localised explication of how gender is played out as a practical accomplishment in men and women's interactions. I examine the way that the interviewer 'positions' participants (Davies & Harré, 1990) and the resulting ideological dilemmas of men's negotiations of this identity (Billig et al., 1988). Wetherell argues that there are often several positions operating within a text, all of which are highly occasioned and potentially inconsistent, and the 'flow of interaction variously troubles and untroubles these positions' (Wetherell, 1998: 400).

Adopting a discursive approach allows a different focus on gender and self-help group identities from previous research. What is distinctive here is a situated focus on how participants (including the researcher) invoke and construct self-help groups and self-help group identities (Potter, 2005). I pay close attention to the way in which, as the interviewer, I position participants as members of a self-help group and thus hold them accountable (Potter, 1996) for that identity. The analysis explicates the significance of men and women's formulations of their involvement in self-help groups.

ANALYSIS AND DISCUSSION

I begin my analysis by noting a surprising phenomenon about the responses that men made to specific questions about their involvement in self-help groups.

Signalling 'trouble'

This study was part of a wider project about gender and health and my interview schedule asked all the participants whether or not they had ever considered going to such a group. As I had contacted this particular group of participants through self-help groups the question seemed somewhat redundant. However, I asked the question anyway, to signal a change of topic and, in doing so, I positioned participants as people who attended a self-help group. One would expect, in light of my access to this group of participants, that this positioning would not be problematic. Indeed, women unproblematically accepted my positioning of them as members of self-help groups (even though a few said that they were encouraged by friends). However, men resisted my positioning of them in this way. Consider Extract 1 below.

Extract 1   **Taken from Individual Interview 9 with Nick[1]**

1.	Sarah	the next question is (.) did you consider going to a testicular
2.		cancer support group when you were ill or after you'd been ill and
3.		obviously [like you did=
4.	Nick	[yeah=well (.) strangely enough no I didn't
5.	Sarah	oh right?
6.	Nick	it was the last thing I wanted
7.	Sarah	oh right?
8.	Nick	erm (.) only (makes puffing out breath noise) (.) if it was
9.		just to get information it was definitely all I wanted =
10.	Sarah	=yeah
11.	Nick	but I didn't (1) (sighs) erm (.) it's not what I wanted=
12.	Sarah	=no
13.	Nick	I didn't want to talk to someone
14.	Sarah	mm
15.	Nick	erm (1) or talk to a group of people
16.	Sarah	mm

In Extract 1 Nick initially overlaps the question about his self-help group involvement with an agreement. However, Nick's reply orients to how this response might not be what the interviewer expected to hear with 'well' and then 'strangely enough' and the stressed 'no I didn't' reinforces this (line 4). Nick continues to resist this self-help group identity by protesting and using the extreme case formulation (Pomerantz, 1987) that it was the 'last' thing he wanted (line 6). An extreme case formulation is a term that Pomerantz used to refer to how people in conversation make a version of some event more effective or persuasive by employing extreme judgments. The researcher's questioning response (line 7) indicates that this was an unusual response that might require further explanation. In the remaining lines of the extract Nick continually displays some kind of interactional trouble (with the puffing in line 8 and the sighing in line 11). Nick constructs involvement of a self-help group as 'not what I wanted' (line 11).

From similar male responses I began to *speculate* that this 'trouble' had something to do with hegemonic masculinity. In contrast to this, women spoke about gaining knowledge from guest speakers, support from fellow members and other activities that one would tend to associate with self-help groups. It is to these typical activities of self-help groups that I now turn.

The importance of attending to stereotypical constructions of self-help groups

Conventional activities associated with such support/self-help groups include advice, support and education. After the topic of self-help groups was initiated, women tended to start talking about their particular group straight away. Occasionally they made some reference to other stereotypical versions of how people might generally view a self-help group (such as sitting around talking about cancer all night), but they appeared to construct their involvement in self-help groups in a way that did not problematise receiving help and support. The next extract is taken from Frances and demonstrates how the women in this data set routinely constructed self-help groups and associated activities.

Extract 2	Taken from Interview 1 with Frances
1. Frances	well that's why (the group) are so useful
2. Sarah	yeah

3.	Frances	'cos you don't want to bore your friends and family with the
4.		details=
5.	Sarah	=no
6.	Frances	and they know what it does (.) I mean most of the (group name) ladies
7.		haven't had chemo
8.	Sarah	right
9.	Frances	there are some (.) we used to talk about what it does to your gut
10.		you know it's not something you normally talk about (laughs)
		[lines omitted]
11.	Frances	so you can only talk about that with a fellow sufferer
12.		(laughter)

In Extract 2 Frances constructs the group as a place that is useful for talking about cancer and the effects that it has on members of the group. Members of the self-help group are positioned as 'fellow sufferers' (line 11) who share experiences (line 9), such as the effects of chemotherapy (lines 6–10), without boring friends or family (line 3).

For this group of women, then, their constructions conform to typical models of self-help groups – they offer a place where you can discuss cancer in a friendly atmosphere. The typical activities of advice and support associated with self-help groups are not problematised. However, when all four men talked about self-help groups they initially set up an exaggerated stereotyped version of this 'conventional' view of self-help groups, and the activities associated with such groups.

Extract 3	**Taken from Individual Interview 17 with Matt**	
1.	Matt	you know (.) but they seemed to be more erm she said er the woman
2.		that run it she had breast cancer and she belonged to the breast
3.		cancer er group and she said it was like a mothers' meeting you
4.		know it was
5.	Sarah	right
6.	Matt	erm (1) you know th there was <u>coffee mornings</u> and <u>stuff like that</u> =
7.	Sarah	=yeah (laughs)
8.	Matt	guys don't er don't want that sort of thing anyway=
9.	Sarah	=no
		[lines omitted]

10.	Matt	and that was how I perceived a self-help group <u>to be</u> that it
11.		was this sort of=
12.	Sarah	=yeah
13.	Matt	you know <u>touchy-feely</u>
14.	Sarah	yeah
15.	Matt	yeah you know [(laughter) they get hold of you and once they
16.	Sarah	[(laughter)
17.	Matt	have you can't <u>escape</u>
18.	Sarah	(laughs) they hug you to death (laughs)
19.	Mattt	yeah yea:ah

In Extract 3 Matt discusses another local self-help group and in doing so builds up a comical portrayal of such groups as being 'like a mother's meeting' (line 3), where there were 'coffee mornings and stuff like that' (line 6). In lines 10 to 19 Matt concludes his narrative of the group by positioning himself as somebody who perceived self-help groups in this way. 'Touchy-feely' (line 13) is the term he draws upon and that such a group would 'get hold of you and once they have you can't escape' (lines 15–17). With the 'you know' (lines 13 and 15), Matt frames the interviewer as aware that self-help groups are parodied in such ways. Furthermore, the interviewer's laughter (lines 16 and 18) and co-construction (line 18) orient to this consensus.

Extract 4:		**Taken from Interview 8 with Cal and Paul**
1.	Paul	I think they expect to come along and find a load of ill people=
2.	Cal	=yeah yeah (laughs)
3.	Paul	[and you know (inaudible due to over talking)
4.	Sarah	[yeah
5.	Cal	[yeah it's er I think it's erm a bit of a I always use this one
6.		but a bit of an alcoholics anonymous thing (2)
7.	Sarah	yeah
8.	Cal	stand up you know my name's Cal Jackson I've had testicular
9.		cancer and then burst into tears and all that sort of thing and
10.		blokes don't like that sort of [thing
11.	Sarah	[they just think I'm not going to do that
12.	Cal	I don't want anybody to cry in front of me or anything like
13.		that=
14.	Sarah	=no
15.	Cal	so they don't want to come along

Immediately before Extract 4 begins Cal and Paul start to discuss the problem of getting men to attend the self-help group that they belong to. Paul says that people might expect to find 'a load of ill people' (line 1). As with Matt, Cal sets up a familiar image of self-help groups: this time it is Alcoholics Anonymous (lines 6–9). Cal dramatises the activities of this type of group by saying, 'stand up you know my name's Cal Jackson I've had testicular cancer and then burst into tears and that sort of thing' (lines 8–9). It appears that the existence of stereotypes is more troubling for men than women because of the potential for being likened to an arguably gendered, stereotypical self-help group member.

Four functions: a matter of identity

Here I analyse the rhetorical functions men achieve by making relevant the exaggerated stereotyped constructions of self-help groups.

First, I concentrate on the types of activities that the men make significant. If we consider Extract 3, the version of a self-help group that Matt spends time building up is described as a 'mothers' meeting' (line 3) and makes the activity of 'coffee mornings and stuff like that' relevant. Similarly, Cal makes the activity of bursting into tears 'and that sort of thing' (Extract 4, line 9) problematic for potential new members. In line 12 of Extract 4, Cal uses active voicing to present newcomers as saying, 'I don't want anybody to cry in front of me or anything like that'. Crying, then, is constructed as a troubled activity. Arguably these activities could be heard as gendered, thus constructing a rejection of them. Moreover, Matt's 'and stuff like that' (Extract 3, line 6); 'that sort of thing' (Matt in Extract 4, line 8) and Cal's 'all that sort of thing' (Extract 4, line 9) and 'anything like that' (Extract 4, line 12) are left unspoken. However, they seem to draw the researcher into their frame of reference as if she should know the type of thing they are referring to.

After setting up these arguably gendered activities, gender is explicitly made relevant in the men's accounts. For instance, with reference to the three-part list (Jefferson, 1990) of 'mothers' meetings', 'coffee mornings' and 'stuff like that', Matt says 'guys don't er guys don't want that sort of thing' (Extract 3, line 8). Jefferson argued that a three-part list is all that is necessary to build up a case as representative. Here, it is a representative list associated with femininity. Matt's use of the membership category of 'guy' appears to be self-inclusive. Similarly, with Cal's phrase 'blokes don't like that sort of thing' (Extract 4, line 10), gender is again made relevant. A second function of these constructions, then, is to foreground gender. Gender is not simply an analyst's category but is also a participant's concern (Stokoe, 2003).

A third rhetorical move that the men make in discussing these activities is to distance themselves from such versions of self-help group identities. For example, we've already seen that 'crying' is heard as a troubled activity, possibly because it is viewed as a gendered activity. The men in the group work hard in their accounts to acknowledge the possible activities associated with self-help groups in a way that distances their identities from these problematic constructions.

Fourth, how other people might perceive the men's self-help group is made relevant in the men's accounts. For example, in line 15 of Extract 4 Cal says, 'so they don't want to come along' (in reference to the troubled activity of crying). The activities that Matt, Paul and Cal orient to are conventionally associated with gender. Their concern here appears to be about the way that self-help groups are perceived, initially by themselves but also for other men who may potentially want to join the group. The reasoning seems to be that if 'blokes' view self-help groups as including feminine qualities and activities then they will be avoided.

The majority of female participants constructed themselves as *gaining* something from self-help groups (support, self-help and information). Thus it appears that stereotypical views of self-help groups are not problematic for the women in the same way that they might be for the men. In contrast, men spent some time dissociating themselves from particular gendered stereotypes of self-help groups. Men's scripting of these stereotypical and comic constructions of self-help groups achieves some important identity work for them such as warding off gendered activities.

Men narrating 'legitimate' involvement in their self-help group

Of course, after resisting the interviewer's research question (which positioned them as attending a self-help group), the men find themselves in an ideological dilemma (Billig *et al.*, 1988). They 'notice' how their resistance to the self-help group identity is at odds with their presence at the group. The interactional business being negotiated by the men in the following narratives displays their orientation to this dilemma.

Extract 5:   Taken from Individual Interview 17 with Matt

1. Matt   but it (1) one of the guys I work
2.   with (.) <u>he</u> went down with it about 18 months after I had it
3. Sarah   mm
4. Matt   and er he went along (1) 'cos he was probably <u>more</u> <u>that</u> sort of
5.   person that=
6. Sarah   =right =
7. Matt   =would do that sort of thing you know
8. Sarah   yeah
9. Matt   I suppose I am now because I went along but (1) I (.) I it (.) when I first
10.   saw it I thought (.) no it's not for me it was (unclear)
11. Sarah   yeah
12. Matt   [then he sort of like
13. Sarah   [so did he tell you about it?
14. Matt   yeah he he rung me up 'cos we weren't working together he'd
15.   left and moved to another company by this point (.) and he rung up
16.   and he said do you want to come along he says ['cos it's really good
17. Sarah   [mm
18. Matt   and erm I sort of had a thought about it (1) I won't go
19.   and then I thought yeah I will so I just went along to one meeting
20.   not expecting a <u>lot</u> erm

In Extract 5 Matt accounts for his change of decision to attend the group through a story about a guy from work who became involved in the group. Matt formulates his friend as 'probably <u>more that</u> sort of person that ... would do that sort of thing you know' (lines 4–7). Interestingly, Matt leaves open the full explanation of what that type of person is. This detail is left for the interviewer to imagine, or is possibly thought to be obvious and in need of no explanation. In the next turn Matt reflexively adds that he is perhaps that type of person now (line 9). In doing so Matt notices an ideological dilemma (Billig *et al.*, 1988). He has positioned himself as not being the type of person who would attend a self help group but his reflexive construction and subsequent

pause and a few hesitations problematise his attendance at the
self-help group. Matt then presents a version of this initial awareness of the group as being 'not for me' (line 10). Following this,
Matt describes how his friend persuaded him to attend the group.
Matt formulates himself as thinking about this invitation and then
deciding 'I won't go' (line 18). However, he then presents a change
of heart with 'then I thought yeah I will so I just went along to *one*
meeting *not expecting a lot*' (lines 19–20; emphasis added). Matt's
narrative of a change of heart is similar to a device identified as
'At first I thought … but then I realized' (Sacks, 1984). This device
is employed to display that speakers are presenting themselves
as having the initial assumptions that any normal person would
have (Woofitt, 2005). By indicating that he only intended to go to
one meeting and didn't expect a lot Matt is doing 'being ordinary'
(Sacks, 1984), or perhaps, in this instance, *being a 'normal' man*.
By using this device Matt protects himself from being seen as the
conventional type of person who attends self-help groups.

Extract 6:   Taken from Individual Interview 9 with Nick

1. Sarah   so what's it like when you've <u>been</u> to the meetings then=
2. Nick   =it suits me 'cos there's not a lot of people <u>there</u>
3. Sarah   yeah
4. Nick   erm (.) you know 'cos <u>I'm not one for</u> (.) you know er
maybe the
5.   stereotypical [erm you know view of self-help groups
[we all get
6. Sarah   [(laughs) [yeah
7. Nick   round in a circle and start crying and feel sorry for yourself
8. Sarah   mm right=
9. Nick   = I mean I'm not into that=
10. Sarah   =no=
[Lines omitted]
11. Nick   erm (.) I probably didn't consider too much somebody
coming at to
12.   the meeting after I started and talking to them and <u>how
useful I would</u>
13.   <u>be</u> [but just getting involved and perhaps <u>sharing</u> in
some of the
14. Sarah   [mm
15. Nick   good things that Cal and the others are doing
16. Sarah   mm mm
17. Nick   erm so you know and and feeling that you know <u>I ought
to put</u>

18.		something back in =
19.	Sarah	=right
		[Lines omitted]
20.	Nick	=YES that's right for me it's about saving lives
21.	Sarah	yeah
22.	Nick	it's about stopping people dying of cancer
23.	Sarah	mm
24.	Nick	for me
25.	Sarah	mm yeah
26.	Nick	ultimately 'cos (.) that's why you talk about it=
27.	Sarah	=yeah

In the above extract Nick makes relevant the activities associated with stereotypical self-help groups and distances himself from the problematic activity of crying and feeling sorry for yourself (lines 2–9). Later in his narrative Nick constructs a realisation that he could be potentially useful to newcomers attending the group (lines 11–18). Nick proceeds to build up his membership of the group, *and thus his identity*, around giving something to the group rather than being in receipt of something from the group. He constructs his reason for attending the group to be concerned with saving lives and stopping people dying of cancer (lines 20–26) and engages in constructing a positive self-help group identity, warding off other potentially problematic identities (such as being in receipt of support).

DISCUSSION

In this study the management of self-help group identity appeared to be more troubled for men than women. First, I noted how men appeared resistant to the way that the interviewer positioned them as members of self-help groups. Next, I described both men and women oriented to stereotypical views of self-help groups, but only the men problematised these gendered stereotypes. Women's accounts of their involvement in their self-help group were organised around the notion of receiving help, whereas men constructed themselves as offering help. The men discursively negotiated what they viewed as 'legitimate' reasons to be engaged in self-help groups as including being able to help save lives, giving advice about testicular cancer and changing the treatment of patients.

My focus on the discursive construction of masculinity made it possible to rethink the link between masculinity and engagement in self-help groups. Adamsen *et al.* (2001) suggested that action-oriented support groups appeal to male cancer patients as a result of gendered coping styles. There may be some truth in this. However, Adamsen *et al.* based their claims on a group that was pre-determined to be active by health professionals. In contrast to this, the men and women in the above data sets have set up and defined their self-help groups themselves. I suggest that Adamsen *et al.*'s findings do not adequately capture the complexity of the issue. Although there may be some currency in the notion that men prefer action-oriented approaches, my analysis in this chapter suggests discussions about a 'preference for action' may be linked more to the presentation of a hegemonic masculine identity than to a preference for action. Gender and health researchers often rush to the conclusion that men and women are different and that one of the reasons for these differences is that they cope differently. Contrary to this position, I am resisting the suggestion that the ways that the men and women in my sample discuss their involvement in self-help groups reflects some innate gendered difference that can be generalised to all men and women. Instead, I suggest that the discursive climate in which this group of men exist places restrictions on potential performances of masculinity. By employing the methods of discursive psychology I have been able to unpack the complexity of this performativity. Furthermore, by incorporating the accounts of women into the analysis I can begin to consider what is specific about masculinity.

The presentation of identity had a material consequence for the members of the self-help group I interviewed – they changed the name of their group from 'testicular cancer self-help group' to a new title, which omitted the troubling 'self-help' concept. This has implications for health promotion. First, the name of self-help groups should be carefully considered, especially if they are to attract men. Second, perhaps health education campaigns need to consider targeting men in ways that appeal or even conform to what we could describe as hegemonic masculine ideals (such as bravado, humour or discretion). Gough and Conner (2006) also raise the issue of what could be referred to as 'gender-specific' health promotion in response to their study about men's eating practices. They argue that barriers to healthy eating can be linked to conventional masculinities which specify autonomous decision-making over obedience to authority.

The above analysis was part of a much larger project about gender and health and, as a consequence, there are a number of limitations to the study. First, the analysis only focuses on a small number of participants. Therefore, it is not possible to make grandiose claims about gender differences in orientations to self-help groups from this data, or indeed from the theoretical position employed. However, there is a pervasive gendered pattern across my data set and future research would benefit from pursuing this line of investigation. A second problem lies in the design of the research and the use of interview data. Future research would benefit from studying self-help group identities *in situ* so that analysis could focus on the site where such identities are produced in interaction rather than being limited to a discussion of men and women's narratives of self-presentation. In interviewing men and women about gender and health I could easily be criticised for bringing my own concerns to the analytic procedure. Whilst this is undoubtedly true, I believe that my close attention to the fine-grained mechanics of discourse have allowed me to demonstrate that gender is also a real concern for the participants.

Attending self-help groups may benefit men's health but it could be argued, based on this study, that being a member of a self-help group is potentially a troubled identity for men. To construct a sense of 'legitimacy' of attendance to such groups this group of men carefully negotiated their identity. I urge future researchers in this area to consider this notion of performativity in more detail. I would also urge those working in the area of health promotion to take into account how men are represented and targeted in their campaigns.

NOTE

1 The form of notation used in this chapter is a simplified version of the transcription notation developed by Gail Jefferson.

REFERENCES

Adamsen, L., Rasmussen, J. & Pedersen, I.S. (2001) 'Brothers in arms': how men with cancer experience a sense of comradeship through group intervention which combines physical activity with information relay. *Journal of Clinical Nursing*, 10: 528–53.

Anderson, B.L. (1992) Psychological intervention for cancer patients to enhance quality of life. *Journal of Clinical Psychology*, 60: 552–68.

Billig, M., Condor, S., Edwards, D., Gane, M., Middleton, D. & Radley, A. (1988) *Ideological Dilemmas: A Social Psychology of Everyday Thinking*. London: Sage.

Bui, L.L., Last, L., Bradley, H., Law, C.H.L., Maier, B.-A. & Smith, A.J. (2002) Interest and participation in support group programmes among patients with colorectal cancer. *Cancer Nursing,* 25(2): 150–7.

Cella, D.F. & Yellen, S. (1993) Cancer support groups: the state of the art. *Cancer Practice,* 1(1): 56–62.

Connell, R.W. (1987) *Gender and Power.* Cambridge: Polity.

Davies, B. & Harré, R. (1990) Positioning: the discursive production of selves. *Journal for the Theory of Social Behaviour,* 20(1): 43–63.

Edwards, D. & Potter, J. (1992) *Discursive Psychology.* London: Sage.

Fitch, M. (2000) Supportive care for cancer patients. *Hospital Quarterly,* 3(4): 39–46.

Frosh, S., Phoenix, A. & Pattman, R. (2002) *Young Masculinities.* Basingstoke: Palgrave Macmillan.

Gough, B. (2006) 'Try to be healthy, but don't forgo your masculinity': deconstructing men's health discourse in the media. *Social Science & Medicine,* 63: 2476–88.

Gough, B. & Conner, M. (2006) Barriers to healthy eating amongst men: a qualitative analysis. *Social Science & Medicine,* 62: 387–95.

Gray, R. & Fitch, M. (2001) Cancer self-help groups are here to stay: issues and challenges for health professionals. *Journal of Palliative Care,* 17(1): 53–8.

Gray, R.E., Fitch, M., Davies, C. &, Phillips, C. (1997) Interviews with men with prostate cancer about their self-help group experience. *Journal of Palliative Care,* 13(1): 15–21.

Gray, R.E., Fitch, M.I., Fergus, K.D., Mykhalovskiy, E. & Church, K. (2002) Hegemonic masculinity and the experience of prostate cancer: a narrative approach. *Journal of Aging and Identity,* 7: 43–62.

Jefferson, G. (1990) List construction as a task and resource. In G. Psathas (ed.), *Interaction Competence.* Washington, DC: University Press of America.

Klemm, P., Hurst, M., Dearholt, S.L. & Trone, S.R. (1999) Cyber solace: gender differences on internet cancer support groups. *Computers in Nursing,* 17: 65–72.

Pomerantz, A.M. (1987) Description in legal settings. In J.R.E. Lee (ed.), *Talk and Social Organisation.* Clevedon: Multilingual Matters.

Potter, J. (1996) *Representing Reality: Discourse, Rhetoric and Social Construction.* London: Sage.

Potter, J. (2005) Making psychology relevant. *Discourse and Society,* 16(5): 739–47.

Sacks, H. (1984) On doing 'being ordinary'. In J.M. Atkinson and J. Heritage (eds), *Structures of Social Action: Studies in Conversation Analysis.* Cambridge: Cambridge University Press.

Stokoe, E. (2003) Doing gender, doing categorization: recent developments in language and gender research. *International Sociolinguistics,* 2(1): 1–12.

Thiel de Bocanegra, H. (1992) Cancer patients' interest in group support programs. *Cancer Nursing,* 15: 347–52.

Vingerhoots, A.J.M. & Heck, G.L. (1990) Gender, coping and psychosomatic symptoms. *Psychological Medicine,* 20(1): 125–35.

Wetherell, M. (1998) Positioning and interpretative repertoires: conversation analysis and post-structuralism in dialogue. *Discourse & Society,* 9(3): 387–412.

Wetherell, M. & Edley, N. (1998) Gender practices: steps in the analysis of men and masculinities. In K. Henwood, C. Griffin & A. Phoenix (eds), *Standpoints and Differences: Essays in the Practice of Feminist Psychology.* London: Sage.

Wooffitt, R. (2005) *Conversation Analysis and Discourse Analysis.* London: Sage.

6 OLDER MEN'S HEALTH: THE ROLE OF MARITAL STATUS AND MASCULINITIES

Kate Davidson and Robert Meadows

INTRODUCTION

From the very onset of interest in gender differences in health it has been claimed that *'women are sicker, but men die quicker'* (Annandale, 2003; emphasis added). Less colloquially put, there exists an 'established wisdom' that within all contemporary industrial societies men have shorter life expectancy than women, although women tend to report more ill health (Morgan *et al.*, 1985). During the 1990s, scholars began to suggest that this paradox arises because 'men's health is profoundly affected by power differences that shape relationships between men and women, women and women, and men and men' (Sabo, 2005: 328). Authors, such as Courtenay (1998, 2000, 2003) and Cameron and Bernardes (1998), identified that men: often see health as women's business and responsibility; know little about their own health; tend to keep quiet about their health problems; tend to deny themselves a self-monitoring role (as health promotion is 'female'); cope less well because of a fear of losing control; and tend to delay seeking help. These social practices, which undermine men's health, were considered tools used to approximate *hegemonic* masculine ideals and to negate the (idealised) feminine norms of health care utilisation and positive health beliefs. In essence, 'doing health' was identified as a form of 'doing gender' (Saltonstall, 1993: 12).

Over recent years, studies have offered a more complex picture while staying true to the fundamentals of this social constructionist approach. For example, Robertson (2003) notes that the historical suggestion that men do not take their health seriously can no longer be sustained (see also Williams, 2003: 60). Rather, men face a dilemma between showing they do not care and realising that they should care and, as a result, caring for health needs to be *legitimised* or explained in some way by men (Robertson, 2003, 2006, 2007). Offering an additional layer of complexity, Watson (2000: 122–42) suggests that men's abdication of personal responsibility to 'look after' themselves is related to the construction of altruistic practice based around pragmatic interpretations. Gough (2006: 2486) also highlights how some men may 'have access to resources which enable "healthy" reinvention of identities and practices while remaining complicit with hegemonic ideals'.

Despite the increased emphasis on differences, complexities and contradictions, older men remain *relatively* absent from empirical work on the links between health and masculine identities (cf. Thompson, 2004). This invisibility is even more surprising when two further things are considered: first, regardless of theoretical starting point, old age is often described as a time when self-identity is challenged. Whitehead (2002: 199), for example, notes that 'as men grow older the authoritative gaze on them changes, and they in turn internalize new subjectivities and sense of self as the years pass, their bodies alter, their health becomes more fragile, their place in the world as men shifts'. Likewise, it is often suggested that hegemonic ideals of manliness emphasise physical strength, (hetero) sexual virility and professional status: facets which are *prima facie* tied into youth.

This is not meant to suggest that all older men will necessarily experience a negative existential crisis. In a study of commonly held images of old men, Thompson (2006) found that old men were favourably described more often than negatively stereotyped. Older men may also remain involved in activities which define them as men, but these activities may take on a different form. For example, a 'busy ethic' may serve as a replacement for an earlier 'work ethic' (Ekerdt 1986; Thompson & Whearty 2004). Rather, it is to suggest that growing older requires men to (re)negotiate masculine identities. Within her study of older adults' experience of Parkinson's Disease, Solimeo (2008) highlights the importance of role continuity in later life. This may be especially difficult for those men who do not have the physical or economic resources available to them or those men who damaged their health in earlier pursuit of dominant masculinities (cf. Calasanti & King, 2005).

Second, older men offer a 'life-course' approach to studies of men's health and masculinities which, in turn, enables investigation into how 'the self of the past is the underpinning of the self of the present' (Thompson & Whearty, 2004: 8). In the UK, for example, a man with a history of working in a professional occupation and living in south-east England is likely to outlive his unskilled manual compatriot in Scotland by some 12 years, with a projected life expectancy of 83 years compared to 71 years (StatBase, 2002; see also Emslie *et al.*, 2004).

A life-course approach also allows for investigation into how life transitions affect the relationship between masculinities, health and embodied experience. For example, it has been suggested that events such as marriage and fatherhood may (unconsciously) draw men 'towards responsible conviviality' (Mullen, 1993: 177) and the successful balancing of control and release or moderation and excess. Somewhat similarly, it is well documented in successive General Household Surveys that older married men report better health than widowed, divorced or never married men (Davidson & Arber, 2003). At all ages over 50, divorced and separated men, followed by widowed men, report poorer health than single or married/cohabiting men (Thomas *et al.*, 1998). Divorced men over the age of 50 report higher rates of smoking and hazardous alcohol intake than other men of their age (Davidson & Arber, 2003) and solo living in old age is associated with an increased likelihood of experiencing loneliness, social isolation and depression (Victor *et al.*, 2002).

This chapter is situated against this backdrop. It examines health, perceptions of well-being and masculinities among older men. Following a discussion of our qualitative methodology, we ask: do (older) men know little about men's health? Do (older) men tend to keep quiet about their health problems? Do (older) men tend to deny themselves a self-monitoring role (as health promotion is 'female')? Throughout the analysis, we keep a firm eye on multiple co-influences and intersections.

METHODS

The data reported here comprise the qualitative component of a larger multi-method research project into the social worlds and health behaviours of older men in south-east England (see

Davidson & Arber, 2004 and Meadows & Davidson, 2006 for a full description of the methodology and its limitations). Eighty-five men over the age of 65 were interviewed, in-depth, in a location of their choice, mostly their own home, in 2001. The sample comprised men who were (a) married/cohabiting (30); (b) widowed (33); (c) divorced/separated (10); and (d) never married (12). The widowed, divorced/separated and never married men are overrepresented in the sample in order to examine the lived experience of lone older men compared to those who were partnered.

The partnership histories of a few of the older men we interviewed were complex. For example, some men had been married more than once: some had been divorced and then widowed, and some had been widowed or divorced and were now cohabiting. The average age of the 85 participants was 75. The divorced/separated men were the youngest group with an average age of 68, and there were none over the age of 76. This contrasts with the oldest group, the widowers, whose average age was 79: 14 out of 33 were 80 or over, with none under 70. Almost all the 85 interviews were carried out by a male researcher who was over the age of 60 and the remainder by the first author.

Older men and 'should care/don't care'

What emerged from the qualitative analysis was a complex picture of health awareness, protection strategies and risk taking. Our interviews with the older men revealed that they knew what was 'good' and what was 'bad' for healthy living. This does not necessarily mean that the men simply put this knowledge into practice. Rather, a system of checks and balances or 'trade-offs' evolved for most of the men:

> Jon (72, married): 'I should walk more. I suppose if I walk round to the post-box round the corner, that's the furthest I go during the week. We try and walk at weekends. … I'm a bad lad, I know. Like for breakfast, I will get up in the morning and probably have two pots of tea, bad for you, eight cups of tea, eight spoonfuls of sugar – wrong. It used to be sixteen, but I have cut the sugar down. Lunch I might have a cheese sandwich, bad for me again. But then I have an evening meal. It would be a cooked meal. Last night it was bacon, tonight it will be a small roast. I like a drink, I probably drink too much, more than what I should do.'

Weather permitting, Jon and his wife went for long afternoon walks at the weekend, by way of compensation for taking little exercise during the week. Jon was not alone in compensating for risky health behaviours. Several said they rarely drank alcohol on Mondays because they would have had several drinks over the weekend. Some only drank alcohol at weekends, or if they were in company, but felt that because they had abstained, they could indulge themselves when drinking socially.

Very few of the men admitted to being 'dangerous' drinkers; that is, drinking more than 50 units of alcohol a week. One was a divorced man who drank wine steadily throughout the interview and offered the interviewer a glass. It was 11 a.m. However, as mentioned above, the men monitored their drinking, generally keeping it to weekends and when in company. The married men drank more regularly, often having a drink with their wife before and at dinner. Like Jon above, a few commented that they probably drank near or over the recommended weekly limit of 28 units. The widowed and single men drank the least often, and divorced men tended to be either abstainers (two were recovering alcoholics) or heavy drinkers.

Most of the men had smoked when younger, and only two (both divorced) continued to smoke more than 40 cigarettes a day. Some of the married men admitted to having a cigar 'on high days and holidays', but most had either ceased, or dramatically cut down their smoking. Interestingly, those who continued to have the occasional cigarette did so in the garden, 'because she [their wife] doesn't like the smell in the house'. This could reflect changing societal attitudes to smoking but also may reflect the wife's disapproval of smoking. Those who had given up or cut down when they were younger tended to do so for economic reasons: taking on a mortgage, having children, and so on. Those who gave up in later years tended to do it for health reasons, and usually on 'doctor's orders'. One gave up after his wife died of cancer, and his daughter had begged him to stop.

These older men's narratives resonate with Robertson's (2006) work on younger men. Robertson (2006: 178) suggests that younger men have to manage two conflicting discourses: 'first that "real" men do not care about health and second, that the pursuit of health is a moral requirement for good citizenship'. As Robertson suggests:

> it is not just caring too much about health that puts hegemonic identity at risk. Not to take enough care with one's health, particularly through indulging in excess, also moves one away from hegemonic ideals. It suggests irresponsibility

and lack of control, which then becomes representative of transgressive (male)
behaviour.

(Robertson, 2006: 184)

Similar to the younger men in Robertson's study, the older men here appear embroiled in a 'should care/don't care' balancing act and are required to tread a path between control and release. For some, the ability to achieve this balancing act later in life seemed worth emphasising; suggesting that it may take on greater importance in situations where other tools and resources used to approximate hegemonic forms of masculinity are not available:

> *I'm one of these lucky people that have suffered good health all my life. ... we are sensible about our eating, we try and do a certain amount of walking exercise each day.*
>
> *(Rory, 84, married)*

> *I have been wonderfully fit, apart from back trouble since my wife died. I don't drink lots of alcohol, I don't smoke, I live a fairly simple lifestyle, a healthy lifestyle.*
>
> *(Peter, 70, widowed)*

With that said, the older men's narratives did highlight 'limits' to their engagement with the 'should care' side of the coin. The narratives also illustrated both deontologically driven and tele-ologically driven changes (cf. Robertson, 2007: 55) which could move men more towards the 'caring' side of the equation. As Robertson (2007) suggests, deontological, or rule-based, drivers include limiting excess in order to be a dutiful partner and father. Teleological drivers include wanting to live long enough to see your child grow older. I shall return to these issues below.

Preventive health and GP use

For many of the men, it was apparent that 'control' literally meant '*self*-control' and that this, in turn, meant that the men rarely engaged with professional preventive health programmes. Only four of the 85 men had ever attended a well-man clinic or blood pressure and cholesterol screening clinics (as opposed to when they were already at a GP or nurse consultation). These were all married and under the age of 75:

> *Well, if there's anything going free to do with health, I usually try to get on to it. I did do a men's health course through Age Concern, a ten-week course about 18 months ago. And if I go to an exhibition somewhere or to an air show, something like that, and they do a blood test and blood pressure, I'll go in and do it, because it's there.*
>
> (Richard, 69, married)

All the men also admitted that they would not go to the doctor unless they absolutely had to; and even then it would be with reluctance.

> *a lot of illnesses, people can deal with it themselves.*
>
> (Gareth, 71, widowed)

> *I don't give in. Even if I felt awful, I wouldn't tell anyone.*
>
> (Paul, 67, divorced)

> *I've always tended to think, well, it's going to go away.*
>
> (Richard, 70, never married)

> *You've just got to get through it.*
>
> (Edward, 71, never married)

This reluctance to engage in help-seeking behaviours was often legitimised through redress to the incompetence of the medical profession. Kevin (75, widowed) said that he would rather go to a veterinary surgeon than a doctor 'after the way they treated my wife'. Even if he had cancer, he said, he would put up with it, rather than seek medical help. Other men stated:

> *most of them [doctors] are a waste of time.*
>
> (Guy, 79, never married)

> *I don't like doctors, I keep as far away from the place ... it's not an exact science, it's about as accurate as weather forecasting – you can quote me on that.*
>
> (Clive, 72, married)

At one level, then, older men's lack of engagement with medical professionals is situated within wider discourses to do with patient's trust. As Trachtenberg *et al.* (2005) suggest, trust in the medical profession is a key predictor in medical care; regardless of age or gender. Yet, at the same time, the men within the present study offered narratives which suggested that their reasons for non-engagement included but went beyond issues to do with trust.

The men constructed frequent use of health care as feminine and seldom use as masculine. For example, Andrew considered illness to show weakness of character. He swam five days a week, a kilometre non-stop on the day of the interview. Despite his scorn for people who succumbed to illness, his wife had had diabetes and died of a heart attack at 49 because she had 'overexerted herself'. But as he said: 'it's a thing for other people', not him. 'Other people' tended to be female. He cited a female neighbour who was 'always at the surgery with something or other' and bothering the GP who should be tending to people who were 'really ill'. Andrew is simultaneously constructing help-seeking behaviours as negative ('bothering GPs') and female. Similarly, other men stated:

> I think it is like, well, ladies will go to the doctors many, many times more than a man. A man says – oh, it came by itself, it will go by itself.
>
> (Jon, 72, married)

The 'frequent use of health care = female' vs. 'the seldom user of health care = male' construction can conflict with the men's attempts to perform the 'should care/don't care' balancing act. As Noone and Stephens (2008) identify in their interview study of seven older men, a third subject position exists which enables men to resolve this dilemma and use health care while maintaining a masculine identity. Noone and Stephens (2008) label this the 'legitimate user position', when men stress that they do not go running to the doctor for everything. Within the present study, the 'legitimate user position' was intrinsically linked to marital status. For example, Jess offered the following:

> My wife has her 'woman' checks. She said to me, 'If I've got to do this, why don't you too?', so I do, just to keep her happy. She says she wants me to be around a long time!
>
> (Jess, 71, married)

Jess echoed the comments from several men who joked that their wives nagged them to go to the GP because they wanted them to be fit and healthy. They also said things like 'she'll only get on at me if I don't', and the underlying impression is that they would not have gone without prompting. As White argues, 'when a man is ill it is normally the female member of the family ... who sanctions the illness behaviour' (2001: 19). For men, this can be a means of legitimising visits to a doctor (Robertson 2003, 2007); as it paradoxically reinforces the notion that health care is women's concern.

The complexities involved with men's constructions of health and health-care utilisation, the balancing of masculine identities and the moral requirement to be good citizens did find some of the men in 'incompatible subject positions' (cf. Noone & Stephens, 2008). This was especially the case with those men who did become embroiled within the health-care system and were in regular contact with health professionals. Below I discuss two types of scenarios found within the interview, and men's responses to them: 'routine compliance' and 'falling to pieces'.

Routine compliance

Several of the men said they never or rarely went to their GP, yet on further probing, they talked about having had major surgery – heart (usually bypass), or cancer (usually prostate) – which required monitoring and follow-up with checks and/or medication, quarterly or annually. The men who reported these visits did not see them as 'sickness' consultations and tended not count them as 'going to the doctor'. These men were visiting their doctors only on a 'routine compliance' basis: because they were requested to attend, rather than having instigated the consultation themselves:

> They tell you to come back, you have to see them once a year, and he sort of puts the old stethoscope on, asks a few questions and tells you to come back next year.
>
> (Jeremy, 68, married)

There was a surprisingly high reportage of asthma, for which the men were prescribed an inhaler after diagnosis. In the UK, it is possible to request a repeat prescription from a surgery without having to see the GP and, while indeed these men were not visiting a doctor, they were still officially undergoing treatment. Although Jon believed that what 'comes by itself, goes by itself', he took regular medication for his asthma, but did not view this as 'treatment' because he felt in control of his condition. 'I am asthmatic I try not to suffer from it ... and being an asthmatic what I try to do is, although I do have it, I try not to suffer.'

Falling to pieces

About a fifth of the men, mostly widowers, reported poor health and were in regular contact with health professionals. They suffered from a variety of serious conditions including cardiovascular disease, diabetes, cancer (prostate and bowel) and musculo-skeletal disease. A few of these men had been ill for several years, but most said that the onset of their illness had been relatively recent. Some men reported that they had been 'fine' until 'X' number of years ago and then 'everything started to go wrong'. We termed this phenomenon 'domino pathologies' whereby the man went to the doctor with one condition and on further investigation, other conditions were diagnosed, including high blood pressure, high cholesterol, other cardio-pulmonary abnormalities, enlarged prostate, chronic liver and kidney disease, and so on.

The older the man, the closer the dominos and the quicker the tumble into multiple conditions. As reported above, the widowed men represented the oldest group in the sample and were the most likely to be in poor health. According to Fries's (1980) compression of morbidity theory, people are most ill in the final two years of their life, whatever age they die. It was therefore expected that this group of men, who were likely to have been older than their spouse and had outlived her, would have poor health after her death. However, our analysis revealed that although there were similarities in narratives about the 'domino pathologies' within the sample of men with poor health, the widowers presented with a different pattern. For the widowed men who had cared for an ailing spouse, analysis showed that the 'X' number of years ago almost always coincided with the death of their wife:

> I'm now 81 and I'm in poor health, very poor health. Up until the age of 75, I was going fine and then I had a serious cancer operation. After that, everything seemed to break down.
>
> (Forrest, widowed)

Forrest had been widowed six years previously. His wife had a long-term illness which required 24-hour care and he was diagnosed with cancer of the prostate three months after her death. He was one of the eight widowers who had cared for a sick spouse and reported poor or deteriorating health soon after her death. The prevailing theme through the narratives was that these men could not afford to be ill while nursing their wife because of their caring responsibilities. It was as if they could only give themselves permission to be ill once the caring role ceased. The widowed men, then, appeared to offer a 'should care/*can't* care' history. They had suppressed, ignored or denied signs and symptoms of ill health which would normally have prompted them (or be prompted) to seek medical attention.

Only four married men were in very poor health, and were looked after by their wife. Of particular interest here, these men's narratives seemed to reflect (and perpetuate) the relationship between masculinities and health-care utilisation discussed above. Whatever pathway was followed to get professional help, many of these men felt that going to the doctor in the first place was the start of their deterioration in health, rather than identification of pre-existing conditions. Further emphasising the complexity of the 'should care/don't care' balancing acts, these married men appear to be suggesting that seeking help (and thus 'caring' too much) was the root cause of their problem.

For example, Sean (75) had 'always led a very active life'. He had been in the Air Force and since going into 'civvy street', he had taken a job as an insurance salesman, 'out on the road', and had enjoyed walking and gardening:

> *I went into hospital at the end of January and had an operation for a heart bypass and a heart valve replacement, both of which were successful and I never had time to worry about them. But during the course of being in the hospital I picked up a hospital bug, and that laid me low and everything I have had since has been post- operative problem, due to this hospital bug.*

Somewhat similarly, Randy (66) had a stroke six months previously while he was in hospital for a cataract operation. The operation was not carried out and he was eventually discharged. He is awaiting a new surgery date for his eyes and at the time of the interview, was unable to see or walk:

> *It's since I've had this, all these problems. Having this stroke and other bits and pieces added to it just in general. I can't get around.*

When asked if there had been anything wrong before he went into hospital, Randy admitted that his 'legs had been bad' and got very swollen at times, but still insisted things started going wrong in the hospital. Because his eyesight had been failing for some years, he had ceased driving and both he and his wife were dependent on their daughter, who lived nearby, for transport.

Discussion

When asked about diet, physical activity, smoking and alcohol consumption, all the men were aware of what was 'good', for them, and the likelihood of ill health resulting from risk behaviours. We could surmise that older men are aware of health promotion information, but, similar to other groups in society, they do not always adhere to advice. Like Robertson's (2007) younger men, the older men within this study were embroiled in a 'should care/don't care' balancing act.

The 'should care' part of these scale seemed very much focused on *self*-care, control and rejecting (medical) interference. Dominant themes within the older men's narratives included a lack of respect and trust for the medical profession and a belief that medics should only be 'bothered' with serious ailments. The older men in this study did not want to be seen to 'give in' to sickness. The men interviewed admitted to postponing making a doctor's appointment until they were very sick. They then have negative associations with the doctor, who they only see when they are in pain, or feel very unwell and importantly, who may give them bad news about their health.

In essence, alongside 'should care/don't care', the men held firm that regular use of health care was feminine and seldom use was masculine. Positioning the two together could cause contradictions and complexities. As in Noone and Stephens's (2008) study, this was resolved through the existence of several other subject positions. The men suggested that they remained reluctant to engage with health professionals until they felt they could no longer resist the persuasion, as Jess said, 'just to keep her happy', or 'she'll only get on at me if I don't'. This phenomenon has been termed the 'nag and drag syndrome' (personal communication) whereby women, after repeated suggestions, eventually wear down the opposition and the men comply. Similarly, several of the men discussed quitting smoking because of children's wishes. This again, echoes research on younger men. Robertson (2007) states how there is a deontological and teleological drive which moves men towards the 'control' end of the balancing act. To be a good, dutiful partner and father requires limiting excess; just as the desire to be there for a child as it grows older does. Much of these changes occur unconsciously and as part of a 'logic of practice'.

This 'legitimate user' position (cf. Noone & Stephens, 2008) illustrates the importance of marital status. Older men who live without women are more likely to lack the health-protective support experienced by partnered men. They are also more likely to have reduced informal social networks since these too are most frequently generated and maintained by women throughout the life course (Scott & Wenger, 1995). The married men were more likely to report continuing good health, and the widowers, as the oldest group, were more likely to report deteriorating health and regular contact with their GP.

Other attempts at successful 'subject positioning' could be seen in those men who had ill health and who were regularly engaging with health professionals. They also attempted to frame their situation in terms synonymous with 'should care/don't care' and seldom use. For example, the prevailing theme through several of the widowed men's narratives was that these men could not afford to be ill while nursing their wife because of their caring responsibilities. Here then, the 'should care' component (that the pursuit of health is a moral requirement for good citizenship) is mitigated by a 'can't care' component (an equally moral requirement to care for one's sick wife).

As men age they may encounter new (masculinity) discourses which are positive in nature (e.g. 'wise old man'). Within the present study, men did discuss some 'compensations' associated with growing older. Those with grandchildren valued the relationship they had with them, often a better and closer one than that with their own children when they were so busy being the family breadwinner. Also, the erosion of men's role as breadwinner has been theorised to result in an increase in the capacity for a less self-serving, more caring style of interacting with others (e.g. Gutmann, 1987). Many spoke of more contented, less conflictual relationships with their wife than when they were younger.

Yet, within the present study the older men's discussions of their health remained framed similarly to younger men's. Contradicting the idea that hegemonic ideals vary through the life course (cf. Robertson, 2007), our findings suggest that older men 'strive to achieve masculinity with similar meanings to those of younger men' (Meadows & Davidson, 2006; Solimeo, 2008: 42), and that they remain structurally situated within the same dominant ideology/discourse as younger men.

Recent UK policy initiatives have been a response to growing awareness of the importance of health maintenance in later life on individual, institutional and societal levels. In early 2008, the government announced that everyone between the ages of 40 and 75 should receive a health check every 10 years for cardiovascular disease, diabetes and kidney disease (Department of Health, 2008). The programme is to be called the Vascular Disease Risk Factor Assessment and Management Programme (Lister, 2008). In this way it is hoped that early detection and treatment will prevent up to 9,500 heart attacks and strokes a year, and annually save 2,000 lives (Department of Health, 2008). The programme is targeted at the whole population, but men are likely to be the greater beneficiaries, since it is these diseases which give men the highest morbidity and mortality rates. The screening is likely to be carried out 'opportunistically' as well as by GP request, with some patients checked when they come for other reasons (Lister, 2008). Although the programme is to be very much welcomed, our findings indicate that it will be accessed principally by married men, persuaded by their spouse, and the widowed men who may have health professional input for bereavement care, or encouraged by adult daughters or nieces to attend. For older men who have had little or no 'ongoing contact' with health professionals (unlike women) in their life course, it seems unlikely that they will turn to the health sector when they reach later life.

It is important to recognise that the customary approach to health improvement has been to target individuals, but less attention has been paid to addressing the broad determinants of older men's health behaviours. These include biological, social, cultural and economic factors that influence men's choices of health-protective strategies and social practices. This holistic approach needs to take into account the socially constructed roles that shape masculinity and femininity throughout the life course that are compounded by economic and cultural influences.

REFERENCES

Annandale, E. (2003) Gender differences in health. In S. Taylor & D. Field (eds), *Sociology of Health and Health Care* (3rd edn). Oxford: Blackwell, pp. 81–97.

Calasanti, T. & King, N. (2005) Firming the floppy penis: age, class and gender relations in the lives of old men. *Men and Masculinities*, 8:1: 3–23.

Cameron, E. & Bernardes, J. (1998) Gender and disadvantage in health: men's health for a change. *Sociology of Health & Illness*, 20(5): 673–93.

Courtenay, W. H. (1998) College men's health: an overview and call to action. *Journal of American College Health*, 46(6): 279–90.

Courtenay, W. H. (2000) Constructions of masculinity and their influence on men's well-being: a theory of gender and health. *Social Science & Medicine*, 50: 1385–1401.

Courtenay, W. H. (2003) Key determinants of the health and well being of men and boys. *International Journal of Men's Health*, 1 January.

Davidson, K. (2001) Late life widowhood, selfishness and new partnership choices: a gendered perspective. *Ageing & Society*, 21(3): 297–317.

Davidson, K. & Arber, S. (2003) Older men's health: a lifecourse issue? *Men's Health Journal* 2(3): 72–5.

Davidson, K. & Arber, S. (2004) Older men, their health behaviours and partnership status. In A. Walker and C. Hennessy (eds), *Growing Older: Quality of Life in Old Age*. Maidenhead: Open University Press and McGraw Hill, pp. 127–48.

Department of Health (2008) Vascular checks will prevent thousands of heart attacks and strokes. http://www.dh.gov.uk/en/News/Recentstories/DH_083836, accessed 1 April 2008.

Ekerdt, D.J. (1986) The busy ethic: moral continuity between work and retirement. *The Gerontologist*, 26, 239–44.

Emslie C., Hunt, K. & O'Brien, R. (2004) Masculinities in older men: a qualitative study in the West of Scotland. *Journal of Men's Studies*, 12: 207–26.

Fries, J. (1980) Aging, natural death and the compression of morbidity. *New England Journal of Medicine*, 303(3): 130–5.

Gough, B. (2006) 'Try to be healthy but don't forgo your masculinity': deconstructing men's health discourse in the media. *Social Science & Medicine*, 63(9): 2476–88.

Gutmann, D. (1987) *Reclaimed Powers: Towards a New Psychology of Men and Women in Later Life*. New York: Basic Books.

Lister, S. (2008) NHS burden to be cut by heart tests for the over 40s. *Times Online*. http://www.timesonline.co.uk/tol/news/uk/health/article739105.ece, accessed 1 April 2008.

Meadows, R. & Davidson, K. (2006) Maintaining manliness in late life: hegemonic masculinities and emphasized femininities. In T. M. Calasanti & K. F. Slevin, *Age Matters: Realigning Feminist Thinking*. London: Routledge, pp. 295–311.

Morgan, M, Calnan, M. & Manning, N. (1985) *Sociological Approaches to Health and Medicine*. London: Routledge.

Mullen, K. (1993) *A Healthy Balance: Glaswegian Men talking about Health, Tobacco and Alcohol.* Aldershot: Avebury.

Noone, J., H. & Stephens, C. (2008) Men, masculine identities, and health care utilisation. *Sociology of Health and Illness,* 30(5): 711–25.

Robertson, S. (2003) Men managing health. *Men's Health Journal,* 2(4): 111–13.

Robertson, S. (2006) 'Not living life in too much of an excess': lay men understanding health and well-being. *Health,* 10, 175–89.

Robertson, S. (2007) *Understanding Men and Health: Masculinities, Identity and Well-Being.* Maidenhead: McGraw Hill and Open University Press.

Sabo, D. (2005) The study of masculinities and men's health: an overview. In M. S Kimmel, J. Hearn & R. W. Connell (eds), *Handbook of Studies on Men and Masculinities.* London: Sage.

Saltonstall, R (1993) Healthy bodies, social bodies: men's and women's concepts and practices of health in everyday life. *Social Science & Medicine,* 36(1): 7–14.

Scott, A. & Wenger, G. C. (1995) Gender and social support networks in later life. In S. Arber & J. Ginn (eds), *Connecting Gender and Ageing: A Sociological Approach.* Buckingham: Open University Press, pp. 158–72.

Solimeo, S. (2008) Sex and gender in older adults' experience of Parkinson's Disease, *Journal of Gerontology Series B: Psychological Sciences and Social Sciences,* 63: S42–48.

StatBase (2002) Population: age, sex and legal marital status, 1971 onwards (England and Wales): Population Trends 109. http://www.statistics.gov.uk/STATBASE/xsdataset.asp?vlnk=5753, accessed 1 April 2008.

Thomas, M., Walker, A., Wilmot, A. & Bennett, N. (1998) *Living in Britain: Results from the 1996 General Household Survey.* London: Stationery Office.

Thompson, E. H. (2004) Guest editorial. *Journal of Men's Studies,* 13(1): 1–4.

Thompson, E. H. (2006) Images of old men's masculinity: still a man? *Sex Roles,* 55: 633–48.

Thompson, E. H. & Whearty, P. M. (2004) Older men's social participation: the importance of masculinity ideology. *Journal of Men's Studies,* 13(1), 5–24.

Trachtenberg, F., Dugan, E. & Hall, M. A. (2005) How patients' trust relates to their involvement in medical care: trust in the medical profession is associated with greater willingness to seek care and follow recommendations. *Journal of Family Practice,* 554(4): 344–52.

Victor, C., Scambler, S., Shah, S., Cook, D., Harris, T., Rink, E. & de Wilde, S. (2002) Has loneliness amongst older people increased? An investigation into variations between cohorts. *Ageing & Society,* 22(5): 585–97.

Watson, J. (2000) *Male Bodies: Health, Culture and Identity.* Buckingham: Open University Press.

White, A. (2001) How men respond to illness. *Men's Health Journal,* 1(1): 18–19.

Whitehead, S.M. (2002) *Men and Masculinities: Key Themes and New Directions.* Cambridge: Polity.

Williams, S.J. (2003) *Medicine and the Body.* London: Sage.

7 PROMOTING 'MASCULINITY' OVER HEALTH: A CRITICAL ANALYSIS OF MEN'S HEALTH PROMOTION WITH PARTICULAR REFERENCE TO AN OBESITY REDUCTION 'MANUAL'

Brendan Gough

INTRODUCTION

There is widespread (but not total) consensus that the state of men's health has reached crisis proportions (White, 2006). For example, men on average die five years younger than women and are overrepresented in statistics on heart disease and non-gendered cancers (see White & Cash, 2003). Most commentators point to 'hegemonic masculinity' as a significant factor here (Connell, 1995; Courtenay, 2000). Briefly, hegemonic masculinities refer to gender ideals which predominate in a given cultural context at any one time which specify hierarchical relations between men, and between men and women. In most Western countries, for example, competitive sport is defined as a heterosexual, masculine domain which subordinates and marginalises women and gay men. In the arena of health, hegemonic masculine practices such as excessive alcohol intake, risk-taking and a penchant for red meat are linked to poor health outcomes such as cirrhosis of the liver, physical injury and bowel cancer (see Courtenay, 2000; White, 2002). Moreover, the whole arena of health is commonly perceived as 'feminine' such that men are portrayed as naïve about their bodies and reluctant to engage with health services (see Courtenay, 2000; Lee & Owens, 2002).

There is now considerable effort on the part of health promotion agencies to engage men in healthier lifestyles. For example, recent UK initiatives have included health professionals visiting places men occupy, such as barbers, pubs, betting shops and workplaces (e.g. Baker, 2001; Banks, 2004).

Apart from such open-ended interventions, there are examples of projects which target specific groups of 'vulnerable' men (e.g. unemployed men) and/or specific health problems (e.g. alcoholism) (e.g. Kierans & Wainwright, 2006). Of particular relevance to men's health, but also resonant more generally, is the contemporary obesity 'epidemic', commonly depicted as a health 'time bomb' in the mass media (see Gough, 2007). It is now routinely claimed that obesity is linked to all manner of serious conditions, from diabetes to infertility and cancer (e.g. Chambers & Wakley, 2002; Men's Health Forum, 2005).[1] Men who fall into medically defined obese and overweight categories can be classed as an especially problematic group since men in general delay reporting symptoms until a disease such as heart disease or cancer has advanced (e.g. Kapur et al., 2004).

Apart from the stigma of being 'fat', 'masculine' ideals about stoicism, endurance of pain and perceived invulnerability may well inhibit men from seeking help early. Conversely, the ubiquitous images of 'six-pack' men with slim but muscular physiques present an obviously challenging ideal of contemporary masculinity for this group, an 'Adonis complex' (Pope et al., 2000) which in some cases may lead to psychological problems (see Grogan & Richards, 2002). Now, health promotion interventions are starting to prioritise 'obese' men (and women), such as the 'HGV Man' manual (Banks, 2005), designed to facilitate weight loss and healthy living, and the subject of analysis here.

The analysis which follows can be situated within a paradigm termed 'critical health psychology', which is predicated on a critique of mainstream psychology and an affinity with other social science disciplines such as sociology (Murray, 2004). With this field, conventional health promotion interventions, often informed by psychological models such as the theory of reasoned action/planned behaviour (see Conner & Norman, 1996), are interrogated on a number of grounds. For example, responsibility for changing behaviour is firmly located with individual subjects who are expected to modify their lifestyles in 'appropriate' and 'rational' ways, as highlighted in health promotion literature and by health practitioners (see Marks, 2002). Hence the social context in which people lead (often complex) lives is erased, and the emotions which are invested in particular health practices are overlooked (Stainton-Rogers, 1991; Rise, 2002).

Critical, qualitative research can help contextualise and illuminate the ostensibly unhealthy activities in which individuals and groups engage. In relation to gay men, for example, Flowers et al. (1997) provide a useful insight into why some gay men reject the use of condoms and risk sexually transmitted diseases (STDs) – his participants rationalise 'unsafe' sex as a sign of commitment in long-term loving relationships. In addition, the work of Monaghan (2005, 2006, 2007) and others (Campos, 2004; Gard & Wright, 2005) has contributed to an evolving literature on 'critical obesity studies' which questions the often dramatic claims made about the dire health consequences of excessive weight and obesity by challenging the medical evidence, critiquing standard measures of obesity (e.g. Body Mass Index) and gathering accounts from ordinary 'fat' people which trouble medical discourses and celebrate larger bodies.

This chapter is an attempt to develop a more detailed critique of men's health promotion by applying techniques from discourse analysis to one text in depth. Other work situated broadly within the social psychology of health has similarly analysed men's health promotion texts, especially those provided by national newspapers (e.g. Lyons & Willott, 1999; Gough, 2006, 2007), as well as texts devoted to specific conditions, such as prostate cancer (Clarke, 1999) and male infertility (Gannon et al., 2004).

The text in question is the *HGV Man Manual* aimed at overweight and obese men (as defined by the medical concept of Body Mass Index) in the UK, and is part of a series of 'man manuals' designed to engage men in healthy living (other titles include 'Man', 'Cancer', 'Baby', 'Sex', 'Woman'). When I first encountered these texts, I was struck by the blatant deployment of stereotypes about men and masculinity evident in the concept of a 'man manual' per se and then in the content of each text. I was then taken with a brief critique of the series by Scott-Samuel (2006), which argued that the masculinities advertised were, ironically, associated with deleterious health outcomes for men and women worldwide. For example, men's presumed detachment from their bodies, conveyed by the car metaphor, can mean a lack of insight in and care of the body, resulting in serious illness which impacts on men and their families. However, there is much more scope to examine the texts in question in order to consider how this drive to improve men's health may in fact be thwarted by an allegiance to hegemonic constructions of masculinity. I have selected the text on obesity for intensive analysis because of the huge public concern in the UK and other Western countries about the supposedly dire health consequences of obesity, and because of the particular vulnerability of 'fat blokes' in an age of media-inspired male objectification (see Gill *et al.*, 2005).

METHOD

The text

The *HGV Man* text, as with other texts in the 'Man' series, is sponsored by Haynes (UK) car manuals, and consciously adopts the recognised style and format of these manuals.[2] Indeed, the inside cover of the HGV Man text depicts examples of car manuals and previous editions of the 'Man' series ('Man', 'Cancer', 'Baby', 'Sex', 'Woman'), emphasising family resemblance and continuity of the brand. The front cover is dominated by an image of a large man superimposed by a thinner figure with some male organs and joints represented by mechanistic devices, e.g. a steering wheel and dashboard for the brain; a pressure gauge for the heart. In the background, photographs of 25 men are presented – face and shoulders only. The title *HGV Man* is positioned on the top left-hand corner of the front page, with the Haynes logo on the top right-hand side. The subtitle is located underneath the title: *Reducing all large sizes; all shapes and colours*, followed by the legend: 'Haynes Owners Workshop Manual'. Below the central image the aim of the text is advertised: 'The practical guide to healthy weight loss'. At the bottom right-hand corner we are informed that 50 pence are donated to the Men's Health Forum with each copy sold. The contents page on the inside features eight chapter titles:

1. Right fuel?
2. Losing weight

3. Exercise
4. Nutrition, water and weight control
5. Going for an 'MOT' (how a trip to the doctor can help you achieve your weight-loss goals)
6. Avoidable medical problems
7. Eating disorders and men
8. Life father, like son?

This list of chapter titles is preceded by a list of sponsors and the author's introduction and acknowledgements, and is followed by nine reference sections which mainly provide links to further sources of information, e.g. 'Weight on the web'; 'Ask your pharmacist'; 'Contacts'.

Approach to analysis

I came to this text with some preconceptions. The 'manual' format struck me as generally rather grating and patronising, and I was puzzled by its apparent popularity. Based partly on my previous analyses of printed media discourses on men's health, I also expected uncritical endorsement of masculinised interests and activities, such as (obviously) driving and maintaining cars, sport and beer-drinking. I was determined, however, to remain open-minded when delving into the text itself, and to examine in detail both the modes of masculinity being foregrounded and the ways in which these were deployed. In discourse analytic terms (see Wetherell, 1998), I was interested in discursive resources (e.g. 'masculinity is bad for your health') and discursive practices (e.g. using 'nature' to explain men's health practices).

In practice, I read through the text a number of times, making notes about possible themes and links to the literature. In so doing, I personally learned a lot about men's health, and the following analysis is not designed to dismiss the content per se, but to identify and discuss the culturally available discourses which help structure the text. After reading through the text several times, I then examined each page in a detailed, line-by-line way, and formally generated a multitude of low-level categories in the style of grounded theory (Glaser & Strauss, 1967). Periodically I would make links between categories, forming clusters of 'superordinate' categories. Following a series of revisions to the category system, I arrived at a reduced number of superordinate categories. I then shifted into discourse analysis mode (see Parker, 1994), where I contextualised these categories in relation to culturally established discourses of masculinity. I also paid attention to how these discourses were constructed and warranted in the text (see Wetherell, 1998). Finally, I considered the implications of the emerging analysis for men's health promotion.

ANALYSIS

In scrutinising this text, I was struck by some parallels in both style and content with mass-market men's magazines such as *Men's Health* and *Loaded*. For example, frequent references to beer, football and cars and a playful, joshing style were in evidence, as is the case in men's magazines (see Benwell, 2004; Stibbe, 2004). Thus the key theme of the analysis below revolves around the maintenance of hegemonic masculinities in the text, a tendency which, in the context of health promotion, is questioned here, since hegemonic masculinities are often associated with unhealthy practices (Connell, 1995; Courtenay, 2000).

In general, a narrow repertoire of rather predictable 'masculine' metaphors and male-dominated domains are invoked to render (feminised) health promotion more palatable for men. The obvious metaphor deployed within the car manual format is man as machine, where the male body is defined and illustrated as a car throughout the text. The irony here, I will argue, is that such a mechanistic depiction of the male body reproduces the hegemonic image of the hard, impenetrable exterior which men treat as an object to be worked upon – not a source of 'softness' or vulnerability. The focus is thus on activities that can be performed on the body to enhance well-being while material on the experience of being overweight and the concomitant emotional and interpersonal difficulties is glossed over. Further discourses are deployed in the text which reinforce traditional (unhealthy) masculinities, such as the rational actor (solving problems) and public persona (at work or in the pub) – subjects who 'do' healthy (diets, exercise), but in a 'masculine' way. Being a 'fat' man is also presented as normal, as the next section illustrates.

Deproblematising the (fat) male subject

Although obesity and related health problems are lamented in the text, great care is taken not to address (overweight) male readers as irresponsible or weak, thus protecting their 'masculinity'. Throughout the text, obese and overweight men are not problematised directly or personally, but via reference to medical statistics and societal changes. For example, various 'fat facts' are presented in different chapters, such as:

Did you know?

– Obese men are 33% more likely to die from cancer than men of healthy weight
– 30,000 deaths a year are directly attributable to obesity.
– 800,000 prescriptions of obesity drugs costs £36 M annually ...
(1.3, i.e. Chapter 1, page 3)

The 'HGV' men reading such statistics may well be comforted that they 'are not alone' (1.5). There is also a prominent insert on the advantages of being fat:

> *In some cultures, being fat is valued – and is even a life saver. For example, life on the isolated pacific island of Nauru is traditionally hard. The inhabitants scraped a living from agriculture and fishing, but the soil is poor and droughts common, so they frequently starved. Being fat allowed them to survive the famines, so the islanders admired big, fat people. Nauruan girls even went on diets to fatten them.*
>
> *(4.2)*

Such stories provide a distraction from the main thrust of the material on the reputed dangers of obesity. The problem is also constructed as general rather than (or as well as) individual. Social changes are invoked to situate the problem outside individuals. For example, a section on physical activity pronounces:

> *The human body evolved for movement. This century has seen us do everything we can to remove the need for movement from our lives. The combustion engine has taken away much of the need for walking from A to B. We invented moving staircases to make it easier for us to climb. Power tools, household appliances, lifts and the like all make for an easier life, but at the expense of our physical fitness. Two million years of evolutionary history, fine-tuning the human body to run, chase, hunt, fish, carry and climb have been overturned in just one century ... This, together with an abundance*

*of high-calorie, cheap food, is the reason why, as a nation, we're all getting
so fat.*

(3.2)

This is an interesting segment which suggests a nostalgia for the
active (masculine?) lives of our 'cavemen ancestors', while also
recognising technological advances. While there is an embedded historical association between masculinity and science and
technology, primacy is accorded to an earlier, more primal masculinity predicated on hunting and gathering. Thus the 'natural'
orientation of 'man' towards elemental activity has been erased
by recent history, and 'we' are all implicated in the development
of sedentary lifestyles. It is the 'nation' which is becoming obese,
not individuals – individuals are not to blame. A section on the
poor health of truckers, for example, is careful to emphasise limited opportunities and facilities rather than, say, the unhealthy
'choices' made by these men. The authors of a report into the
issue are quoted as follows: 'It was striking how many of the men
[truckers] we spoke to were worried about the impact it [work]
was having on them but, because of the nature of the work, didn't
know what they could do to look after themselves any better' (1.1).

The men are first presented as concerned about their health,
and their lack of knowledge about protecting their health is
clearly attributed to deleterious working conditions rather than
personal weakness.

Another way in which large or unhealthy men are constructed is
in terms of 'normal' male habits such as drinking beer and eating
junk food. For example, advice on losing weight suggests: 'To burn
off the pint-and-a-half you had at lunchtime (260 kcal) you need to
walk 5 km in an hour. To lose a couple of chocolate bars (600 kcal)
you'd need to run 9 km in an hour. And to get rid of your mum's
roast dinner and sponge pudding (1440 kcal) you have to exercise
as hard as a competitive cross-country skier for an hour' (4.2).

Here, the male reader is directly addressed ('you') and
assumed to casually indulge in a range of routine daily vices,
namely alcohol consumption, unhealthy snacks and traditional
hearty meals – a 'three-part list' (Jefferson, 1990) which helps
normalise this scenario. Every reader is implicated and the activities mentioned are construed as common and normative. In the
age of the 'tyranny of the six pack' (Gill *et al.*, 2000; Labre, 2005)
and a widely touted 'obesity epidemic' (repeatedly underlined in

the HGV text, e.g. 4.2), obesity is commonly construed as personal weakness, lack of discipline, and even immoral. Such attributions could be construed as an attack on masculine identity, but this language is avoided in the text. The mix of scientific ('kcal') and 'matey' ('pint-an-a-half') discourse works to lend authority and urgency to the problem on the one hand and to normalise the situation for individual men on the other.

In constructing the unhealthy male, then, great care is taken not to undermine masculine identities. This is facilitated by a pervasive informal style, continual use of humour, and an explicit agenda to avoid authoritarian health education. The assumption seems to be that men will be deterred by standard health promotion initiatives which (implicitly) lament unhealthy activities and prescribe major lifestyle changes. Consider the very first and last lines in the author's introduction to the text (0.11): 'Make no mistake, this HGV Man Manual is not another pontificating, finger-pointing bit of heavy goods. It is more than just a book about men and weight. It is fun, functional and totally fat-free ... What you won't find is patronising pap to put you off living. Read on to lighten the load. Keep on Truckin'.'

So, there is a distancing from other moralistic health promotion texts which make untenable demands of male readers. Instead, the HGV manual is constructed as something special, a text which is both light-hearted and effective, designed to appeal directly to men and their lives. As such, men's 'masculinity' (independence, rationality, etc.) need not be threatened, since the implication is that men will not respond to heavy-handed imperatives ('Don't you just hate relying on others for anything?!, 8.10). Hegemonic masculinity is also preserved through the predominant image of the male body as a car-like entity, as I now discuss.

The male body as machine

The male body as machine is obviously heralded by the recognised car-manual format which is actually published and distributed by the company who specialise in car and motorcycle manuals in the UK (Haynes). The male machine is supported by various cartoons running through the text, for example a man consuming petrol ('which is the right fuel?', 1.5), man as a car ('think of the bloodstream as a motorway ...', 4.13) etc. And as one would expect with the car-manual format, various car-related metaphors are used to describe the male body and its functions. The focus of Chapter 2, for example, is on losing weight and is framed by subheadings like 'Understanding what's under your bonnet' (2.1) and 'Your weight-loss journey' (2.2). The latter section refers to the following stages (following the Stages of Change Model by Prochaska *et al.*, 1992):

– leaving the car in the garage (the pre-contemplation stage)
– getting in the driver's seat (the contemplation stage)
– starting the engine (the preparation stage)
– releasing the handbrake (the action stage)
– reaching your destination (the maintenance stage)
– the return journey (the relapse stage) (2.2)

Clearly, the male body is an 'engine' which needs to be worked on in a logical, sequential way and treated with care in order to function optimally. The emphasis is on thinking ([pre-] contemplation) and action ('get your motor running', 3.2) rather than feelings. Similar language is used throughout the text, such as:

'Do you spend as much time looking after yourself, thinking about what fuel you need to perform well and how best to recharge your batteries as you do your vehicle?

'Do you service and MOT your body and mind and consider what will keep you mentally and physically in peak condition?'

(2.5)

In this extract, all men are assumed to be car owners and interested in car maintenance. Both body and mind are considered here, both constructed as objects to be manipulated for better performance. Food is configured as fuel, a standard 'masculine' theme (see Roos *et al.*, 2001). The language of the heart, the possibility of vulnerability and emotional experience generally, is omitted.

Men are also closely associated with other machines or equipment, such as bicycles (photograph, 3.19; cartoon, 8.17) gym equipment (3.9; 8.16), and gadgets ('to help you get fit', 3.27). A 'logbook' is also provided to record 'maintenance and servicing intervals' (4.20) where items such as diet, alcohol intake and weight and blood pressure are assessed periodically over a year in order to monitor progress. This endeavour is clearly governed by medical science indices whereby all variables are operationalised and rendered measurable (diet in calories, alcohol in units per week, etc.) – there is no scope to record the *experience* of going through a weight-loss programme on such a structured 'objective' tool.

The whole of Chapter 5 ('Going for an MOT: How a trip to the doctor's can help you achieve your weight-loss goals') is modelled on man as machine, with the following sections covered:

Assessing your fuel intake (5.1)

The importance of regular maintenance checks (5.2)

Visiting an 'obesity bodyshop' (5.4)

Getting a jump start (5.5)

The (male) doctor is thus a mechanic (illustrated in a cartoon, 5.2), with the power to diagnose problems and fix what is damaged. The prevailing image, again, is of the male as a disembodied machine amenable to objective assessment and corrective surgery from a qualified professional. Yet, there is brief mention of potential emotional issues, tucked away in one short paragraph, entitled 'Tell your doctor or practice nurse how being fat is making you feel':

> *Although it may seem difficult at first, it will help your doctor or nurse if you could explain how being fat makes you feel. Be as open and honest as you can. Don't just describe the physical repercussions (e.g. shortness of breath, frequent tiredness), also try to describe how you feel on an emotional level (e.g. does your weight problem leave you feeling depressed, do you comfort eat?)*
>
> *(5.3)*

This invitation to self-disclose thus departs from the overarching man–machine analogy, and is couched rather tentatively ('it may seem difficult at first'; 'if you could'; '… as you can'; 'try to …'), implying that men might feel uncomfortable in the (feminine) world of emotion. Given the fleeting and cautious quality of this appeal, and in light of the utter dominance of the machine metaphor which disavows emotions and prioritises observable 'habits', 'activities' and measurements, it is likely that the importance of personal experience and emotions is lost.

In this section I have presented only some of the main instances of the man–machine metaphor, but want to stress here its pervasiveness throughout the text. The next section concentrates on another dominant motif: the rational actor.

The male mind: rational and autonomous

Although the male body as machine may be worked on by the professional doctor-mechanic, it is not surprising that this health promotion text mainly calls upon men themselves to perform the required body work. But this appeal is framed in particular ways which construct men as rational, independent actors capable of achieving clearly defined goals. The above-cited stages of the 'weight-loss journey' (2.2) conjure up an image of the lone hero struggling to progress through a clear and logical sequence towards attaining weight reduction. Again, there is little scope for the feminised domains of emotion (except, perhaps, some aggression) and help-seeking, which is generally presented as a last resort (indeed, other people apart from health professionals are largely absent in men's self-contained, depopulated universe).

Throughout the text, men are assumed or encouraged to be sensible, realistic and balanced:

> *If you want to lose weight, it is important that you have realistic expectations. (2.1)*

> *Men know Diets with a capital D don't work. (2.3)*

> *The most important thing about motivation is goal setting. (2.6)*

In order to lose weight and become healthy, psychological discourse is deployed which presents men as in control of their own destiny:

> *Make your decisions based on logical discussion with yourself rather than allowing them to be a fait accompli. (2.5)*

> *Knowing how powerful your thoughts are will give you another tool for your kitbag. (2.6)*

> *Weight management is just a matter of choosing the right foods. (4.11)*

Health promotion discourse generally has been decried as individualistic and overly rational (see Murray, 2004; Crossley, 2000), encouraging individuals to be responsible for their health and responsive to education. In doing so, this discourse reproduces hegemonic masculinity, since men are conventionally regarded as autonomous, instrumental (task-centred) and thoughtful, whereas women are assumed to be interdependent, expressive (people-oriented) and embodied (Segal, 1990). It is hardly surprising, then, that the male readers of the *HGV Man Manual* are positioned as 'powerful', achievement-oriented and logical. The theme of 'goal-setting' is of course familiar in other 'masculine' domains such as sport, management and the military (see Knoppers & Anthonissen, 2005). Indeed, these three domains are variously invoked to help promote individual performance. For example, men are invited to 'plan your attack' (3.23) in order to increase physical exercise, to 'fight the insulin resistance' (4.12), and are advised that 'the key to winning the war of terror on fat is to boost your metabolic rate through diet and regular exercise' (4.14). In addition, the Football Association is cited in the context of advice on water intake (4.10) and nutrition (4.18). Indeed, the first page proper (0.11) features a half-page photograph of five England footballers advertising the manual and an acknowledgement below of the Football Association's 'encouragement and assistance'. The world of work is also presented at various points to highlight the problems and possibilities of healthy activities. For example, the case of policemen (4.10–4.16) is used to illustrate the health risks posed by a desk job with little opportunity for exercise of healthy eating combined with a male-centred drinking culture. Whatever the 'masculine' context or discourse, men are consistently advised to use their logical minds and inner strength to achieve a healthy weight.

DISCUSSION

The three interlocking themes highlighted above work to promote hegemonic masculinities as well as healthy lifestyles for men. First, overweight men and their habits (e.g. drinking beer, eating meat) are normalised, responsibility for obesity and ill health is placed elsewhere (e.g. in 'society'), and only small adjustments to men's practices are suggested. Secondly, the prevailing metaphor of the car fixes the male body as a machine to

be scrutinised and mended, reinforcing the traditional detachment of men from their bodies, and by extension, the world of
emotions and vulnerability. Thirdly, the male mind is presented
as rational and divorced from other minds/people as men are
called upon to follow logical steps in the pathway towards attaining prized goals such as weight loss. Although clearly designed
to appeal to men and promote healthier living, this reliance on
hegemonic masculinities is arguably counter-productive, given
the established link between 'male' attributes (e.g. perceived
invulnerability, emotional detachment) and poor health (e.g.
heart disease, suicidality) (Courtenay, 2000). There seems to be
an acceptance of 'how men are' (Seymour-Smith *et al.*, 2002)
and a reluctance to challenge masculinity too much, hence the
emphasis on modest change delivered in a 'friendly' format.

Men who fall within the medical categories of 'overweight' and
'obese' (as measured by the Body Mass Index), the target readers of *HGV Man*, are bound to feel at least slightly vulnerable
in the light of the constantly rehearsed obesity epidemic and
also the 'tyranny of the six-pack' (Gill *et al.*, 2000) which now
saturates popular culture, including magazines like *Men's Health*
(Stibbe, 2004). Yet the text does not provide a therapeutic discourse wherein men can position themselves as feeling subjects,
needing to talk to professionals about their self-image in the
light of their outcast obese status. Instead, stature as an indicator of masculinity is implicitly upheld, and 'solutions' to obesity
focus on the masculinised body and mind, and on male-centred
practices, but not the feminised heart. This is not to uncritically
advocate psychotherapeutic interventions for 'obese' men, but to
highlight the lack of space in which such men can articulate the
impact that their status has on their sense of self, and relationships with others. Health promotion which perpetuates a narrow
range of male stereotypes, while appealing to some men, may
well encourage ultimately health-defeating practices, and may
deter many men from engaging with their health in the first
place (Scott-Samuel, 2006).

Although we should recognise the importance of men's well-
being and welcome the increasing awareness of men's health
issues generally, UK initiatives such as the 'Man' manuals
which recycle a restricted range of masculinised symbols and
practices – and which focus mainly on individual rather than
societal changes – should be treated with some caution. Further

efforts are required which incorporate a greater array of masculine identities and activities and which acknowledge the ostensibly changing nature of masculinities in contemporary consumer societies. For example, men are increasingly incorporated as body-conscious consumers, investing in a range of health and beauty products – although even here masculinised symbols such as the muscular physique dominate advertising (Labre, 2005). There is now a sophisticated social science literature on men and masculinities (Segal, 1990; Connell, 1995; Edley & Wetherell, 1995; Connell & Messerschmidt, 2005) which could inform men's health promotion.

The analysis presented here could be extended to other men's health promotion texts in the UK, including the other 'Man' manuals published by Haynes. It would also be fruitful to compare UK materials with other men's health promotion texts produced in other national contexts, since masculinities can vary cross-culturally (see Connell & Messerschmidt, 2005). Also, other high-profile initiatives could be analysed, such as the use of footballers and male celebrities to educate men about testicular cancer, and outreach work where health professionals deliver advice to men in their communities. Men's health promotion has also been presented through the mass media, for example national newspaper supplements, and these texts have received some critical attention (Coyle & Sykes, 1998; Lyons & Willott, 1999). Indeed, more recent analyses of men's health discourse in national print media chimes with the themes presented here, suggesting that certain hegemonic masculinities prevail across diverse men's health initiatives (Gough, 2006, 2007). In sum, the analysis here suggests that hegemonic masculinities dominate health promotion aimed at obese men and that, as a result, men's poor health status may, ironically, may be compromised. More work is required to interrogate other men's health projects so that, ultimately, effective interventions can be designed which reflect multiple, changing masculinities, and which move beyond the mere 'education' of individuals towards collective, material initiatives.

NOTES

1 Medical sociologists have recently disputed the validity of the obesity 'crisis', questioning forms of measurement such as the Body Mass Index (BMI) and

the putative role of obesity in contributing directly to serious illnesses (see Gard & Wright, 2005; Monaghan, 2005).

2 Details of the book can be found at http://www.haynes.co.uk/webapp/wcs/ stores/servlet/BookFeature_HGVManualView?langId=-1&storeId=10001& catalogId=10001).

References

Baker, P. (2001) The state of men's health. Men's Health Journal, 1(1): 6–7.

Banks, I. (2004) New models of providing men with health care. Journal of Men's Health & Gender, 1(2–3): 155–8.

Banks, I. (2005) The HGV Man Manual. Yeovil: Haynes Publishing.

Benwell, B. (2004) Ironic discourse: evasive masculinity in men's lifestyle magazines, Men and Masculinities, 7(1): 3–21.

Campos, P. (2004) The Obesity Myth: Why America's Obsession with Weight is Hazardous to your Health. New York: Gotham Books.

Chambers, R. & Wakley, G. (2002) Obesity and Overweight Matters in Primary Care. Oxford: Radcliffe Medical Press.

Clarke, J.N. (1999) Prostate cancer's hegemonic masculinity in select print mass media depictions (1974–1995). Health Communication, 11(1): 59–74.

Connell, R.W. (1995) Masculinities. Cambridge: Polity.

Connell, R.W. & Messerschmidt, J.W. (2005) Hegemonic masculinity: rethinking the concept. Gender & Society, 19(6): 829–59.

Conner, M.T. & Norman, P. (eds) (1996) Predicting Health Behaviour: Research and Practice with Social Cognition Models. Buckingham: Open University Press.

Courtenay, W. (2000) Constructions of masculinity and their influence on men's well-being: a theory of gender and health. Social Science & Medicine, 50, 1385–1401.

Coyle, A. & Sykes, C. (1998) Troubled men and threatening women: the construction of crisis in male mental health. Feminism & Psychology, 8: 263–84.

Crossley, M.L. (2000) Rethinking Health Psychology. Buckingham: Open University Press.

Edley, N. & Wetherell, N. (1995) Men in Perspective: Practice, Power and Identity. Hemel Hempstead: Prentice Hall and Harvester Wheatsheaf.

Flowers, P., Smith, J.A., Sheeran, P. & Beail, N. (1997) Health and romance: understanding unprotected sex in relationships between gay men. British Journal of Health Psychology, 2, 73–86.

Gannon, K., Glover, L. & Abel, P. (2004) Masculinity, infertility, stigma and media reports. Social Science & Medicine, 59: 1169–75.

Gard, M. & Wright, J. (2005) The Obesity Epidemic. London: Routledge.

Gill, R., Henwood, K. & McLean, C. (2000) The tyranny of the six pack: men talk about idealized images of the male body in popular culture. In C. Squire (ed.), Culture in Psychology. London: Routledge.

Gill, R., Henwood, K. & McLean, C. (2005) Body projects and the regulation of normative masculinity. Body & Society, 11(1): 37–62.

Glaser, B. & Strauss, A. (1967) The Discovery of Grounded Theory. New York: Aldine.

Gough, B. (2006) 'Try to be healthy, but don't forgo your masculinity': deconstructing men's health discourse in the media. *Social Science & Medicine*, 63: 2476–88.

Gough, B. (2007) 'Real men don't diet': an analysis of contemporary newspaper representations of men, food and health. *Social Science & Medicine*, 64(2), 326–37.

Grogan, S. & Richards, H. (2002) Body image: focus groups with men and boys. *Men and Masculinities*, 4(3): 219–32.

Jefferson, G. (1990) List construction as a task and resource. In G. Psathas (ed.), *Interaction Competence*. Washington, DC: University Press of America.

Kapur, N., Hunt, I., Lunt, M., McBeth, J., Creed, F. & MacFarlane, G. (2004) Psychosocial and illness related predictors of consultation rates in primary care – a cohort study. *Psychological Medicine*, 34: 719–28.

Kierans, K. & Wainwright, A. (2006) *Preston Men's Health Evaluation*. Liverpool: Liverpool John Moores University Centre for Public Health.

Knoppers, A. & Anthonissen, A. (2005) Male athletic and managerial masculinities: congruencies in discursive practices? *Journal of Gender Studies*, 14(2): 123–35.

Labre, M.P. (2005) Burn fat, build muscle: a content analysis of *Men's Health* and *Men's Fitness*. *International Journal of Men's Health*, 4(2): 187–200.

Lee, C. & Owens, R.G. (2002) *The Psychology of Men's Health*. Buckingham: Open University Press.

Lyons, A. & Willott, S. (1999) From suet pudding to superhero: representations of men's health for women. *Health*, 3(3): 283–302.

Marks, D.F. (2002) Freedom, power and responsibility: contrasting approaches to health psychology. *Journal of Health Psychology*, 7: 5–19.

Men's Health Forum (2005) *Hazardous waist? Tackling the epidemic of excess weight in men*. London: Men's Health Forum, www.menshealthforum.org.uk.

Monaghan, L. (2005) Discussion piece: a critical take on the obesity debate. *Social Theory & Health*, 3: 302–14.

Monaghan, L. (2006) Weighty words: expanding and embodying the accounts framework. *Social Theory & Health* 4: 128–67.

Monaghan, L. (2007) McDonaldizing men's bodies? Slimming, associated irrationalities and resistances. *Body & Society*, 13(2): 67–93.

Murray, M. (ed.) (2004) *Critical Health Psychology*. Basingstoke: Palgrave Macmillan.

Parker, I. (1994) Discourse analysis. In P. Banister, E. Burman, I. Parker, M. Taylor & C. Tindall (eds), *Qualitative Methods in Psychology: A Research Guide*. Buckingham: Open University Press.

Pope, H., Phillips, K. & Olivardia, R. (2000) *The Adonis Complex: The Secret Crisis of Male Body Obsession*. New York: Simon & Schuster.

Prochaska, J., DiClemente, C. & Norcross, J. (1992) In search of how people change. *American Psychologist*, 47: 1102–14.

Rise, J. (2002) Review of P. Norman, C. Abraham & M. Conner (eds), *Understanding and Changing Health Behaviour: From Beliefs to Self-regulation*. London: Harwood. *Journal of Health Psychology*, 7: 737–9.

Roos, G., Prattala, R. & Koski, K. (2001) Men, masculinity and food: interviews with carpenters and engineers. *Appetite*, 37: 47–56.

Scott-Samuel, A. (2006) Life in the fast lane?, *Men's Health Forum Magazine*, 9, http://www.menshealthforum.co.uk/userpage1.cfm?item_id=1136.

Segal, L. (1990) *Slow Motion: Changing Masculinities, Changing Men*. London: Virago.

Seymour-Smith, S., Wetherell, M. & Phoenix, A. (2002) 'My wife ordered me to come!': a discursive analysis of doctors' and nurses' accounts of men's use of General Practitioners. *Journal of Health Psychology*, 7(3): 253–67.

Stainton-Rogers, W. (1991) *Explaining Health and Illness: An Exploration of Diversity*. Hemel Hempstead: Harvester Wheatsheaf.

Stibbe, A. (2004) Health and the social construction of masculinity in *Men's Health* magazine. *Men and Masculinities*, 7(1): 31–51.

Wetherell, M. (1998) Positioning and interpretative repertoires: conversation analysis and post-structuralism in dialogue. *Discourse & Society*, 9: 387–412.

Wetherell, M., Taylor, S. & Yeates, S.J. (2001) *Discourse as Data: A Guide to Analysis*. London: Sage.

White, R. (2002) Social and political aspects of men's health. *Health*, 6(3): 267–85.

White, A. (2006) Men's health in the 21st century. *International Journal of Men's Health*, 5(1): 1–17.

White, A. & Cash, K. (2003) *The State of Men's Health Across 17 European Countries*. Brussels: European Men's Health Forum.

Willig, C. (2004) Discourse analysis and health psychology. In M. Murray (ed.), *Critical Health Psychology*. Basingstoke: Palgrave Macmillan.

8 THE HEALTH EXPERIENCES OF AFRICAN-CARIBBEAN AND WHITE WORKING-CLASS FATHERS

Robert Williams

INTRODUCTION

In the UK there is increased interest amongst policy makers and practitioners in 'men's health'. This interest is reflected in a developing body of research that addresses the links between masculinity, or masculinities, and men's experiences of health. However, fathers, who play key roles in facilitating or inhibiting the health and well-being of families and communities, have remained peripheral to this developing body of work. This is in spite of evidence that suggests that health and welfare services find it difficult to engage fathers. For example, a UK study indicated that fathers were 'peripheral' to 'Sure Start' health and welfare initiatives targeted at children and families (Lloyd *et al.*, 2003). Unfortunately, policy regarding families in the UK continues to focus upon women as gatekeepers to family health and welfare, in spite of evidence for the increasing involvement of fathers in the care of children within families in the UK (O'Brien, 2005). A limited policy focus on fathering is compounded by the absence of a coherent focus upon men's gendered health experiences. For example, the 'Choosing Health' (Department of Health, 2004) strategy for health promotion recognised the importance of 'behaviour', 'lifestyle' and 'choice' for the health of men and women, but included no real strategic intention to improve gender sensitivity within health care. This chapter, therefore, reports on a qualitative empirical study with African-Caribbean and white working-class fathers regarding their health beliefs and practices in order to identify implications for future research, policy and practice. The background to the study is initially examined, before methodology, findings, and a discussion of the implications are outlined.

BACKGROUND

The conceptual underpinning of this qualitative study was Connell's (1995, 2005) work regarding masculinities, which was valuable in assisting analysis of African-Caribbean and white working-class fathers' configurations of gender practice. Connell argues that differing configurations of masculinities that may enable or constrain men have their foundation in social inequalities between men and women. However, Connell's work is also invaluable in that his framework also integrates differences in power between groups of men in society. Connell differentiates between differing configurations of practice, and specifically differentiates between a politically and culturally dominant form of hegemonic masculinity with less powerful configurations such as subordinated masculinities (e.g. sexual minorities), and marginalised masculinities (e.g. ethnic minority and poor working-class men).

While there is limited published literature in the UK regarding fathers' gendered experiences of health, there is an emerging literature that attempts to consider the relationships between masculinities and men's health (Moynihan, 1998; Chapple & Ziebland, 2002; Oliffe, 2005; Emslie et al., 2006; Robertson, 2007). Robertson (2007) found that masculinities can enable or constrain men's health beliefs and practices, and that health beliefs were associated with changing masculinities. An earlier investigation, regarding fathers' health experiences, found that health for fathers of diverse ethnic backgrounds may be linked to the need to 'get by' or 'go the distance', that is, health may be necessary for men to remain active as workers and/or fathers in everyday life (Williams, 1999). Watson's (2000) work has also indicated that experiences of 'parenthood', specifically, were associated with men 'letting go' of their bodies, with the body talked about as being constrained by economic and social obligations. This chapter builds on this developing body of work regarding masculinities and health by reporting on men's health experiences as fathers within the life course, with specific analysis of African-Caribbean and white working-class fathers' stories about the meaning of health, the influences upon their health, and regarding their health practices.

METHODOLOGY AND METHODS

The concept of masculinities (after Connell, 1995, 2005) was important in planning this critical and qualitative methodological framework, in the sense that it was necessary to explore, respect and understand fathers' experiences as agents, while at the same time recognising the impact of social structures and materiality on those experiences. Access to the six African-Caribbean and seven white working-class men involved in the study was through purposive sampling, using community contacts in a city within the West Midlands in the UK. The 13 informants were well men (not service users, patients or clients), in paid work, living with a woman partner, living with some (or all) of their children, and living in one locality segmented by areas of deprivation and affluence. Men were recruited as experienced fathers of older children (rather than infants and toddlers), their ages ranging between 27 and 48. Two semi-structured interviews were undertaken with each father, and qualitative data analysis was informed by the work of Mills (1973), Burgess (1984) and Miles and Huberman (1994) in order to seek out contradictions and diversity as well as patterns within the data. Ethical scrutiny was undertaken within a British university, pseudonyms identified by participants and all data cross-checked to ensure anonymity.

FINDINGS

Through the data analysis, four interdependent themes were identified as being of key significance: 'Health as functional capacity', 'Influences on fathers' health', 'Fathers' health practices' and 'Masculinities and fathers' health beliefs and practices'.

Fathers' health as functional capacity

The recurring pattern within fathers' stories regarding the meaning of health was what I have termed 'health as functional capacity'. That is, fathers talked about health as being a capacity that was linked to the perceived obligations of paid work, but also the obligations of fathering. For example, Brandon summarised this point very succinctly:

> For me, personally, good health is not catching colds, ... being able to get up and get out, get to work, and run around with the kids.
> *(Brandon, 'British of Barbadian ancestry', police officer)*

Health for fathers within this study was an asset to allow paid work and fathering to take place without disruption. Similarly, Herzlich (1973) had earlier found that some individuals may conceptualise health as a 'reserve', and Watson (2000) in his research with men, specifically, found that some men talked about health as a 'resource' which allowed men to keep functioning in everyday life. However, health as functional capacity has other dimensions within this study. As Brandon's response above indicates, health is also understood as absence of disease (as Herzlich [1973] also found). Furthermore, some fathers also talked about health involving 'fitness'. 'Fitness' was also framed in functional terms:

> I take some exercise, a bit of running or jogging, we go walking as a couple or as a family. So if I wasn't able to do a bit of hill walking or to run five miles, then I'd say I wasn't fit and probably wouldn't be healthy either. I'd be packing on the pounds again. It's really being fit enough to live the life that I want to live, really. You know ... with my daughter and that ...
> *(Trefor, 'Welsh', social care worker)*

Health as functional capacity, then, allowed fathers to fulfil their perceived obligations within families and workplaces, but fathers' health experiences were mediated by a series of important factors which will now be outlined.

Influences on fathers' health

Racism

Stories of fathers from both groups provided little evidence for a link between their ethnicity and health. One African-Caribbean father referred to the incidence of 'sickle cell' and 'thalassaemia' amongst African-Caribbean people, and another identified climate differences between Jamaica and England as being of significance to him. Regarding racism, only one white father, Trefor, had personally experienced racist prejudice and abuse:

> *I lived in Surrey for 20 years and the racism that I experienced as a Welsh person was usually very overt. I was a 'Welsh cunt' and I've been called that more times than I care to remember, but also the less overt stuff.*
>
> *(Trefor, 'Welsh', social care worker)*

In contrast to the group of white fathers, regarding the possible links between racism and health most African-Caribbean fathers told stories about how they anticipated or experienced prejudice, abuse or discrimination in communities or workplaces For example, Terrence told me:

> *What really annoys me is if you are at the checkout, you are going to pay for something, and you give them money. You put your hand down on the table, and they put their hand down on the money, like that! To avoid touching your hand. So I then look at my hand, or look to see if they do it to someone else. And you will remember it, you have stored it away.*
>
> *(Terrence, 'black and British', production line worker)*

These experiences of marginalisation, and objectification by others, within the stories of African-Caribbean men were often extremely disturbing. Brandon, for example, told me:

> *the job I do is confrontational, and you are going into people's homes and lives. You are going into places where people feel most secure, and in their opinion this is their castle. I come along and I change all those rules. The upshot of this is that the person will go on the defensive, and they will go for you: 'Black bastard!'*
>
> *You get that type of abuse. Because I am a sergeant now, I get the stereotypical 'Who is in charge?'*
>
> *'I am', I say.*
>
> *'You can't be, because you're black!'*
>
> *... When I am not in work I get it less.*
>
> *(Brandon, 'British with Barbadian ancestry', police officer)*

The impact of such experiences was often perceived to be uncertain, with terms like 'stress', 'pressure', 'hassle', or 'battle' being used to describe them. For example, Liam told me:

> *It's like I told you before. You know, when I confronted that racist kid on the bus. It was a hassle, but I needed to be strong. Not fighting, like ... but I couldn't*

back down. I turned round and told him what I thought. It is stress, but you've got to do it … Or they will always do it, won't they? It is stress, just stress.
(Liam, 'black Irish', unemployed building labourer)

The sometimes uncertain or hidden nature of the racism African-Caribbean fathers experienced was compounded by the uncertain impact these stressful experiences had on their health, although Karlsen and Nazroo's (2002) earlier work does suggest that the experience of perceived or anticipated racism may be associated with both physical and mental health problems.

Social class?

Blaxter (1990) found that lay concepts of health may underplay social explanations. Indeed, fathers within this study had little directly to say about the possible influence of their social class background on their health, although the influences of paid work on fathers' health were considerable, as will become clear later in this chapter. One father's story was, however, distinctive:

Health is about stress. There is a reason why you may have to drink every day or why you can't say no, or, if you're overweight, but it really comes down to stress. As a working-class family we can adapt to a different environment. We're immune to a lot of stress. Other families would be stressed out.
(Liam, 'black Irish', unemployed building labourer)

Unlike other fathers interviewed, Liam's exceptional account links together unemployment, social class, the local environment and experiences of stress. No other fathers told stories like this, but paid work was understood as being significant within their health experiences, as will now become clear.

Paid work

While fathers generally did not talk about the links between social class and health, the influence of paid work on their lives was considerable. Earlier work by Jahoda (1982) and Warr (1987) has identified the health benefits, particularly for individuals' mental health, associated with paid employment. For fathers within this study, paid work was certainly a necessary way for men to meet their perceived economic obligations within families, but was also a source of stimulation or social contact or provided a sense of well-being or pleasure, such as 'having a laugh' with other men, or even providing a sense of achievement. For example:

I'm doing things I enjoy at work, keeping fit and getting stimulation by speaking to different people, new students, students from abroad, so you get to know different people, so it's good.

(Paul, African-Caribbean, fitness instructor)

Paid work was also experienced by men as affecting their health in a variety of negative ways. Difficulties within the workplace such as the limited autonomy associated with production-line labour, racism, threats to personal safety and environmental hazards, but also the insecurity of potential unemployment, were experienced by individual men in differing ways, dependent on their occupation, employers and work environment. Tiredness or exhaustion were identified by some men who worked shifts as stressful experiences. Some men talked about the intensity and volume of work in terms of consequences for their physical health. For example, Sylvester worked for a building company, but was a 'subbie', formally a self-employed sub-contracted plasterer. Chronic pain in his right arm and shoulder, influenced by the volume and intensity of his work, began when Sylvester was in his thirties, some 18 years previously:

In my case I start thinking what will it be like in the next ten years? At the moment the worst part of my body is the pain barrier in my arm, you know. Sometimes I cannot sleep at night, and you start thinking will my arm hold up? If I have an easy week it is not so bad ... I don't have to push myself, but you get weeks when you have a job you have to push more and it hurts more.

(Sylvester, 'Jamaican first, and English', plasterer)

While paid work was important in influencing the health of fathers, their stories consistently emphasised the combined influences of both paid work and fathering, which will be considered next.

The combined effects of paid work and fathering

In Williams (2008) it has been reported that the involvement with children by fathers was linked with dynamic forms of masculinity. Here, the specific enjoyment of emotional reciprocity ('love') shared with children was highly valued by all men interviewed. For some fathers involvement with children could also help with, or alleviate stressful work experiences. Involvement with children could also be stimulating, involving teaching or learning with children, or could be creative within play with children. For example, Ron said:

> *But a nice time for me is like tonight, when they all come home. We sit on the set-tee for an hour, all three of us. We will then all watch the television. We will nor-mally all end up shouting and arguing, playing about, or something. But, those times are important, that's what being a father is. Being there for them, and they all say 'Can we have a cuddle, dad? ... if they are a bit upset over something.*
>
> *(Ron, 'British', production-line worker)*

On the other hand, fathering was also associated with more nega-tive health experiences, although the specific difficulties that each father experienced were varied. Some fathers indicated that they had fears about potential threats to children's health or security, while other fathers found it difficult to deal with children's auton-omy (especially as they became young people), or deal with chil-dren's 'behaviour'. For some of the fathers with young children, or fathers working shifts, broken sleep patterns and the associated tiredness or exhaustion were difficult experiences. Sometimes dif-ficulties at home affected work relationships, and sometimes work difficulties, and fathers' irritation or verbal aggression, affected relationships with women and children, as John told me:

> *when you are tired it is very difficult being the sort of parent you want to be really, you want to be a rational and patient, caring person, but sometimes if you are in the wrong frame of mind you may think they are being naughty, but sometimes they are not being naughty. Sometimes that can be quite hard. If you are tired you are not really up to the job are you?*
>
> *(John, 'British and Irish', production-line worker)*

Fathers, as a whole, experienced conflicts or tensions between competing obligations of paid work and family life. Ron, who had separated from his wife shortly after the study began, experienced these tensions in a more intense form than any other father:

> *it's a vicious circle. I mean there are times when I think, I need to pack up work altogether to care for the children on my own so ... That would be great ... I am pinned in to what I am doing now ... The only way my work is good for my family life is the money.*
>
> *(Ron, 'British', production-line worker)*

There is a developing body of research addressing the impli-cations of paid work and caring for the health of women (e.g. Cunningham-Burley *et al.*, 2006), but there is limited evidence about the links between fathering, paid work and health. However, this study's findings do confirm Warin *et al.*'s (1999) research which found that fathers experienced difficulties in dealing with the obligations of both paid work and domestic domains. Watson's (2000) work has also demonstrated that men, including fathers, may experience their bodies as 'fragmenting' over time. Fathers, within this study, were also aware that, over time, they may have gained more body weight, or their body shape had changed, or they may have felt less lithe, less physically strong, less 'fit' than before, or that men talked about experiencing a combination of these changes taken place within the context of fathering and working. Furthermore, the combined affects of paid work and fathering also created a more restricted sense of agency for fathers. Their stories indicate that doing paid work and involvement with children limited their personal autonomy: for some men this involved limited scope for a career or promotion at work, for others their scope for personal development was limited, and for some fathers their social life with friends, or with women partners, had 'slowed down', as some men put it. For example, Sylvester said:

> *Being a parent takes a lot, really. You tend to forget yourself, really. You leave yourself out, really. So you haven't got any independence. You take a little piece here and there. It is not what you would ideally like, but that is the way it is.*
>
> *(Sylvester, 'Jamaican first, and English', plasterer)*

FATHERS' HEALTH PRACTICES: PHYSICAL ACTIVITY AND CONSUMPTION

Fathers within this study were involved in a range of practices which they perceived influenced their health but which they also found pleasurable. Such practices included playing the guitar, nurturing Bonsai trees, walking, jogging, running, boxing, 'working out', football and squash. These activities were talked about as 'healthy' practices, although their involvement in such activities was often constrained by and talked about in contrast with paid work and fathering obligations:

> *Throughout the whole week I try and do a minimum of three hours in the gym …
> I love it. I absolutely love it. Especially because I can see some of the results now, I feel fitter and healthier. I enjoy it and it is a form of release.*
>
> *(Brandon, 'British, of Barbadian ancestry', police officer)*

While Brandon alone talked about physical activity as a form of 'release', most fathers talked about such practices as enjoyable experiences that were different to and distinct from paid work and involvement with children.

All fathers were also involved in transgressive forms of consumption, that is, they broke certain perceived rules which they 'ought' or 'should' not do. Specifically, fathers enjoyed smoking 'fags', or 'binge drinking', or 'going on the beer', or eating 'junk', 'treat' or 'crap' food. For example, Don told me about his experiences in the 'pub':

> *it is my time to go out and have a few beers, and to enjoy myself ... but to go out with independent people and let your hair down with someone who is nothing to do with the family. Or you can go out and discuss things which are complete and utter crap, and it doesn't matter.*
>
> *(Don, 'British', firefighter)*

However, fathers' stories demonstrated that such transgressive practices were linked, for them, to family and paid work constraints. Transgressive consumption helped men relax or alleviate difficult experiences at home or at work. In this sense the ways in which fathers understood health as functional capacity, their restricted sense of agency associated with obligations of paid work and fathering, and transgressive consumption are linked. Health was an asset to allow men to meet the obligations of paid work and family life, paid work and family life constrained men's lives in a variety of ways, and transgressive consumption provided men with some pleasure in living with such constraints.

All fathers talked about how that these forms of transgression may affect their body weight and body definition in terms of diminishing 'fitness', health problems in the future, and conflict for some fathers when 'going on the beer'. Furthermore, while most fathers were certainly reflexive about transgressive consumption, there were contradictions and ongoing ambivalence in stories as well. In fact, findings are consistent with Crawford's (2000) work: Crawford has argued that people may have ambivalent patterns of denying and enjoying the pleasures of consumption. More recently Robertson (2007) has identified a 'don't care'/'should care' dichotomy in men's stories about health. Fathers' stories here also indicated that the experience of fathering was linked to reflexivity about the form, volume and location of transgressive consumption of cigarettes, alcohol and food.

For example, most fathers' consumption of food was influenced by preparing 'healthy' not 'crap' food for children. Furthermore, some men indicated that they had changed, or intended to change, their activities regarding cigarette smoking, drinking alcohol, and food consumption, unsafe car driving, and also the limited amount of physical activity they did, because of their obligations to children. For example, John said:

> *I packed up smoking after the birth of our second child, because I thought I will try and be around for a while now, I made that decision.*
>
> *(John, 'British and Irish', production-line worker)*

For the men within this study both paid work and fathering mediated their stories about health and influenced their health practices. However, what is the association between fathers' health experiences and masculinities?

MASCULINITIES AND FATHERS' HEALTH BELIEFS AND PRACTICES

One of the most surprising findings within this investigation was the evidence for solitary beliefs and practices by fathers regarding health. All fathers indicated that they were involved in solitary ways of thinking, feeling and acting alone in order to prevent the disclosure of their 'weakness' or vulnerability to other people. Fathers would use other practices to attempt prevent disclosure of their vulnerability to others. These practices included containing difficult feelings, rational thinking alone, avoiding seeking others' help, but also transgressive forms of consumption and physical activity. For example, Martin told me:

> *You see, I don't think I could talk to people about my worries about my health. It's not that I am secretive or anything. It's just, like, I do worry, I am a bit scared if I'm honest about it, but I wouldn't tell people about what the stress is like. Well my wife spots it, but she doesn't know about these palpitations and all that. I just gotta deal with it myself.*
>
> *(Martin, 'British', telesales supervisor)*

Martin, like other fathers, did feel vulnerable but the prevention of disclosure of vulnerability was often identified by fathers in this study as a 'strength'. Disclosure of vulnerability may be a 'burden' for women and children which fathers intended to prevent.

Courtenay (2000) has earlier argued that control or denial of vulnerability was linked to hegemonic masculinity in men's stories about health. Within this study, most fathers explained their solitary beliefs and practices by linking such experiences to gender. It is worth focusing on Martin's account once more, to illustrate this point:

> *It is like asking for help. I have never done it. It might be a sign of weakness maybe. Going to back to like the cavemen type of thing, being the leaders .... I hate asking people for help.*
>
> *(Martin, 'British', telesales supervisor)*

O'Brien *et al.* (2005), in their study regarding masculinities and help-seeking, found that ahistorical discourses about masculinity were used by some men to explain inflexible and unchanging practices. In this study, fathers repeatedly explained solitary experiences with reference to men's perceived ancestors, or there was talk about 'primitive' men or 'cavemen', as if aspects of their own experiences were inevitable. Fathers employed essential, ahistorical and hegemonic masculine discourses to explain their solitary experiences.

A narrow view of fathers as stoical, silent or isolated is not, however, borne out by study findings because there was also evidence that fathers were reflexive about their children's, and particularly boys', ongoing or potential solitary experiences. In contrast to the last excerpt above, Martin also told me this story about his relationship with his son:

> *I like to think I am always there for my son, which is quite an important thing. So often you hear about, or read stories . ... a boy who lives around the corner from here actually hung himself because he was being bullied at school, and I keep saying please talk to me, no matter how silly it is, just talk to me. That is quite an important thing because so much seems to be happening at the moment, and with the last year of juniors the pressure will be on him a bit more. Sometimes he seems worried and I ask him what he is worried about and he says nothing ... I don't like to put him under pressure too much.*
>
> *(Martin, 'British', telesales supervisor)*

Fathers' stories also, then, provided evidence of attempts to challenge the solitary or the potentially solitary experiences of children, particularly boys. Within individual fathers' stories and within the data as a whole there are contradictory beliefs and practices: conservative notions about solitariness and masculinity on the one hand, and challenges to such reified notions on the other. If considered alongside the evidence of fathers' reflexivity and change about transgressive forms of consumption, stimulated by their obligations to children, fathers' changing and contradictory forms of masculinity may provide opportunities for research, policy and practice. These issues will be discussed in the final section of this chapter.

DISCUSSION

Connell's (1995, 2005) concept of masculinities helps us understand the power relationships between different groups of men. For this study, evidence indicates that the African-Caribbean fathers, distinctively, were marginalised by experiences of anticipated or perceived racist prejudice, abuse or discrimination, which were significantly stressful experiences with potentially negative implications for their health. However, while there is evidence of hegemonic masculinity within both groups of men's stories, they were all working-class fathers whose health and livelihoods were linked to unequal power relationships with managers and employers within organisations functioning within globalised free-market capitalism. To this extent there was, therefore, also evidence of marginalised configurations of practice.

Evidence presented within this chapter also indicates that men of both ethnic groups thought, felt and acted in solitary ways to prevent disclosure of perceived vulnerability to others. Fathers within the study recurrently associated such solitary experiences with hegemonic forms of masculinity, which was associated with perceived 'strength' rather than 'burdening' others with 'weakness'. However, findings do not confirm stereotypical views about hegemonic men achieving 'strength through silence' (O'Brien et al., 2005), because it is also evident that where men talked about fathering, in particular, changing beliefs about masculinity were evident in men's stories. Fathers were keen to prevent children, and particularly boys, having solitary experiences in the future. Indeed, fathering was also associated within men's stories with reflexivity and changes in their own practices regarding the volume, form and location of transgressive forms of consumption. Hence, transgressive consumption and solitary hegemonic masculine experiences were both challenged by fathers' practices as men living with their children.

Watson's (2000) and Robertson's (2007) earlier work found that men's experiences of masculinity encourage and constrain men's health practices. This chapter builds on this developing work by emphasising that fathers' health experiences are mediated by masculinities, and influenced by tensions between fathering and paid work within the life course. Fathers' beliefs about health as functional capacity were linked with both a restricted sense of agency and transgressive consumption. Health as functional capacity was an asset to allow men to be actively involved in fathering and paid work, but the combined affects of fathering and paid work were also associated with a restricted sense of personal agency for fathers. Men's accounts linked these latter constraints with transgressive forms of consumption, which helped men to enjoy pleasure in living with the obligations of fathering and paid work.

Regarding potential policy implications, it is first worth emphasising that the 'gender duty' within the Equality Bill does make it an explicit responsibility of public-sector organisations in England, Scotland and Wales to take proactive steps to positively promote gender equality for men and women. This policy development does provide potential research and development opportunities, and this study emphasises that fathers of differing ethnic backgrounds may experience health and masculinities in contradictory and unpredictable ways, as Connell (2005) has earlier argued. This latter point means policy development needs gender sensitivity to recognise the heterogeneous ways in which men's configured gender practice takes place, and how this mediates health experiences within the life course. However, public health developments within England are dominated by a new hegemony of individualistic neo-liberal values, with a narrow focus on individual 'behaviour', individual 'lifestyles' and individual 'choice' (see Department of Health, 2004, for example). Findings indicate that the implications of paid work and fathering are particularly important within fathers' health experiences. UK government policies to support a 'work–family balance', to support parents' care for children and to enable increased care leave, paternity or parental leave (Department of Trade and Industry, 2005) are to be welcomed. Nevertheless, it must also be emphasised that awareness by policy makers about how social divisions like gender, racism, ethnicity and social class impact on fathers' health experiences is required if policies and services are to successfully engage fathers, and public health policy and practice can respond to structural factors, as well as agency (often called 'behaviour').

Research priorities within the National Health Service and academia, in England, may well focus on findings presented here about transgressive forms of consumption, which are not unimportant. However, I would emphasise that the ways in which the constraints of hegemonic masculinity were mediated and challenged within men's stories about being a father require attention. A specific research opportunity therefore exists to investigate whether public health activity can help fathers to help boys develop their awareness and skills for improving their gendered health.

REFERENCES

Blaxter, M. (1990) *Health and Lifestyles*. London: Routledge.

Burgess, R. (1984) *In the Field: An Introduction to Field Research*. London: Allen & Unwin.

Chapple, A. & Ziebland, S. (2002) Prostate cancer: embodied experience and perceptions of masculinity. *Sociology of Health and Illness*, 24(6): 820–41.

Connell, R.W. (1995) *Masculinities*. Cambridge: Polity.

Connell, R.W. (2005) *Masculinities* (2nd edn). Cambridge: Polity.

Courtenay, W. (2000) Constructions of masculinity and their influence on men's well-being: a theory of gender and health. *Social Science & Medicine*, 50: 1385–1401.

Crawford, R. (2000) The ritual of health promotion. In S. Williams, J. Gabe & M. Calnan (eds), *Health, Medicine and Society: Key Theories and Future Agendas*. London: Routledge, pp. 219–35.

Cunningham-Burley, S., Backett-Milburn, K. & Kemmer, D. (2006) Constructing health and sickness in the context of motherhood and paid work. *Sociology of Health and Illness*, 28(4): 385–409.

Department of Health (2004) *Choosing Health: Making Healthy Choices Easier*. London: Department of Health.

Department of Trade and Industry (2005) *Work and Families: Choice and Flexibility. A Consultation Document*. London: Department of Trade and Industry.

Emslie, C., Ridge, D., Ziebland, S. & Hunt, K. (2006) Men's accounts of depression: reconstructing or resisting hegemonic masculinity. *Social Science & Medicine*, 62: 2246–57.

Herzlich, C. (1973) *Health and Illness*. London: Academic Press.

Jahoda, M. (1982) *Employment and Unemployment: A Social-Psychological Analysis*. Cambridge: Cambridge University Press.

Karlsen, S. & Nazroo, J. (2002) Agency and structure: the impact of ethnic identity and racism on the health of ethnic minority people. *Sociology of Health & Illness*, 24(1): 1–20.

Lloyd, N., O'Brien, M. & Lewis, C. (2003) *Fathers in Sure Start*. London: University of London Institute for the Study of Children, Families and Social Issues.

Miles, M. & Huberman, A. (1994) *Qualitative Data Analysis: An Extended Sourcebook*. London: Sage.

Mills, C.W. (1973) *The Sociological Imagination*. Harmondsworth: Penguin.

Moynihan, C. (1998) Theories of masculinity. *British Medical Journal*, 317: 1072–5.

O'Brien, M. (2005) *Shared Caring: Bringing Fathers into the Frame*. Manchester: Equal Opportunities Commission.

O'Brien, R., Hunt, K. & Hart, K. (2005) 'It's cavemen stuff: but that is to a certain extent how guys operate': men's accounts of masculinity and help seeking. *Social Science & Medicine*, 61: 503–16.

Oliffe, J. (2005) Constructions of masculinity following prostatectomy-induced impotence. *Social Science & Medicine*, 60: 2249–59.

Robertson, S. (2007) *Understanding Men and Health: Masculinities, Identity and Well-Being*. Maidenhead: Open University Press.

Warin, J., Solomon, Y., Lewis, C. & Langford, W. (1999) *Fathers, Work and Family Life*. London: Family Policy Studies Centre.

Warr, P.B. (1987) *Work, Unemployment and Mental Health*. Oxford: Oxford University Press.

Watson, J. (2000) *Male Bodies: Health, Culture and Identity*. Buckingham: Open University Press.

Williams, R.A. (1999) *Going the Distance: Fathers, Health and Health Visiting*. Reading: University of Reading and Queen's Nursing Institute.

Williams, R.A. (2007) Masculinities, fathering and health: the experiences of African-Caribbean and white working class fathers. *Social Science & Medicine*, 64(2), 338–49.

Williams, R.A. (forthcoming) Masculinities and fathering. *Community, Work and Family*.

Part 3

MEN, MASCULINITIES AND ILLNESS

9 PATHOLOGISING FATHERHOOD: THE CASE OF MALE POST-NATAL DEPRESSION IN BRITAIN

Ellie Lee

INTRODUCTION

This chapter discusses the emergence of male Post-Natal Depression (PND) as a health concern in Britain. Up to the early 1990s, PND was represented as an exclusively female condition. Some, however – including medical professionals, academics and media commentators – now take a different view. PND, they suggest, can affect men, and some argue almost as many men as women are affected (Ballard *et al.*, 1994; Curham, 2000; Matthey *et al.*, 2001; Welford, 2002; Sheringham, 2003; Goodman, 2004; Rawles, 2004; Huang & Warner, 2005).

In recent reporting, the lowest estimate of the proportion of new fathers affected is 4 per cent, with figures of 7 per cent (Coltman, 1998) and 10 per cent (Orvice, 1994) also being suggested. Figures in these instances place the incidence of male PND as somewhat lower than that found in women (estimates of the prevalence of PND in new mothers range from 10 to 70 per cent (Brockington, 1996; Figes, 1998; Dalton & Holton 2001; Wolf, 2001). Yet, other reports about male PND suggest a comparable figure. For example, in 2000 it was reported that 15 per cent of new fathers have PND on the basis of estimates from Australian psychiatrist John Condo (Peterkin, 2000), and in 2004 it was stated that 'as many as one in four new dads suffer from post-natal depression' (Rawles, 2004).

The diagnosis of PND as a male as well as female condition may appear to constitute a move away from an essentialist/biological determinist model of illness that has frequently been deemed problematic by feminists in particular (Oakley 1980; Miles 1991). The labelling of women's experience as 'female disorders' through medical diagnoses including hysteria, pre-menstrual syndrome (PMS) and PND has been the subject of powerful criticism (Tavris, 1992; Figert, 1996; Nicolson, 2000). It has been argued that providing such diagnoses 'reduces women to their biology', making the problems women experience appear to be the result of 'raging hormones' rather than, say, gendered oppression in general and the demands and expectations of the mothering role in particular (Ehrenreich & English, 1973). In conventional accounts of PND, hormonal changes associated with the biology of pregnancy and childbirth have been considered causal. The American Psychiatric Association (2001) argues, for example, that PND is caused by changes in hormones. The category of male PND appears to move away from this model, since it is only when the cause of PND is understood differently i.e. as non-biological in origin, that the illness can be diagnosed in men. The category of male PND requires that the connection be severed between depression and pregnancy and childbirth as primarily biological events.

However, the argument made here is that the ascendance of a non-biological model of PND suggested by the spread of its diagnosis to men does not *in itself* generate a genuine alternative to essentialism (the belief that behaviour can be explained by a single, underlying, causal essence) and its close ally biological determinism (the idea that the best explanation for behaviour is biological and, more specifically, genetic). As I will illustrate, animating almost all discussion of male PND appears to be a highly deterministic account of the problems of contemporary fatherhood, which can be termed 'emotional determinism'. The argument that men should be diagnosed with PND is for this reason, I will argue, best thought of not as an alternative to but a version of an essentialist approach. To discuss this proposition, I take as data claims made about male PND in the public domain between 1992 and 2005 in popular media, medical journals, and on lobby groups' websites. I discuss the claims made therein with reference to three areas of sociological analysis. First, I draw on work about the process of medicalisation. Second, I consider social constructionist accounts of 'the problem of fatherhood'. Third, I situate male PND in relation to an analysis of 'masculinity' and its pathologisation.

In conclusion, I suggest that a central aspect of the emergence of male PND is the validation of the need for professional intervention in child rearing. In this regard, arguably the most important dimension of the emergence of male PND is the associated application of socio-cultural assumptions about mothering to fathering. The idea that mothers cannot be relied upon to rear healthy children without expert 'support' is a well-worn part of the modern construction of motherhood (Hardyment, 2002; Kukla, 2005). While mothers remain the main target of expert messages about child rearing (and are still assumed to be the primary caregivers), child rearing is increasingly considered the responsibility of men as well as women. The emergence of male PND suggests that that the advocacy of equality in this area of social life entails the construction of both sexes as similarly in need of emotional management as parents.

GENDER, MEDICALISATION AND MALE PND

A funny thing happened on the way to theorizing medicalization: men's bodies were ignored ... with the exception of a few scattered but important pieces ... medicalization research has focused on genderless or female bodies.

(Rosenfeld & Faircloth, 2006: 1)

It was during the 1970s that theories of 'medicalisation' – the process through which the language of medicine comes to dominate explanations for social problems – were first developed (Conrad, 1992). Gender rapidly became discussed as part of this theorisation of the construction of social problems, and as Rosenfeld and Faircloth indicate, above, the view was strongly espoused that medicalisation affects women to a far greater degree than men. In her oft-quoted contribution on the subject, Riessman (1983) wrote that while men's lives had been medicalised in some areas – for example through 'stress management programmes targeting male executives' – most 'routine areas' of men's lives had not be constructed in medical terms. In particular, she indicated that 'men's psychological lives have not been subjected to scrutiny nearly to the degree that women's emotions have been studied' (1983: 15), and argued that, in contrast, women were the 'main targets' of medicalisation processes. Of the twentieth century she stated: 'A plethora of female conditions has come to be ... reconceptualized as illnesses', citing as examples sexual dysfunctions, pregnancy care, fertility, menopause, ageing, teenage pregnancy, wife-battering, PMS and weight (1983: 9–10).

Recent years, however, have seen attention paid to what has been termed elsewhere 'the medicalization of masculinity' (Rosenfeld & Faircloth, 2006). This attention results from recognition that accounts of medicalisation have rarely discussed representations of male experience, but that a strong case can be made that it is necessary to do so. The picture painted in accounts such as that from Riessman do not match with emergent health concerns which have men's lives and experiences at their centre, including impotence and its treatment with Viagra, baldness, attention deficit hyperactivity disorder (ADHD), and post-traumatic stress disorder (PTSD) in the military (see chapters in Rosenfeld and Faircloth 2006 for discussion of these subjects). It is also the case that health concerns deemed previously female-only, including some of those cited by Riessman, above, have crossed the gender divide. It has been claimed, for example, that the menopause affects men in middle age as well as women. Anorexia and deliberate self-harm, psychological problems associated most often with females, are now represented as disorders that affect more and more young men (BBC News Online 2003b, 2004). Men are now considered to be at risk from breast cancer, and concern about cancer in men in general has been actively encouraged (Lee & Frayn, 2008). This chapter provides a further example of this trend, discussing, as it does, male PND.

A further aspect of recent theorisation of medicalisation is also relevant. Recent accounts of medicalisation processes have argued that a model that places medicine and medical professionals at its centre – so called 'medical imperialism' – is outdated, if it was ever correct (Furedi, 2006). In relation to gender, this insight suggests that notions of patriarchal medicine as the main driver of medicalisation, leading to the pathologising of women's experiences to a greater degree than men's, should be viewed as questionable. Rather, it suggests that medicalisation is now reflective of wider socio-cultural trends, not just simply an expansion by (male) medical professionals of their domain of influence. For this reason, medicalisation now tends be viewed as characterised by a process that involves claimsmaking by a wide range of social actors, including most strikingly, lay actors (Conrad & Potter, 2000; Furedi, 2006, 2008). This point appears to hold true for male

PND: a range of social actors including lay groups, journalists, counsellors and agony aunts, as well as psychiatrists, have all promoted the idea that it will help some contemporary fathers to be diagnosed with PND.

Some psychiatrists and psychologists have thus strongly endorsed the idea that men, as well as women, get PND (Matthey *et al.*, 2001), with one arguing that 'The post-natal depression found in women four to six weeks after delivery is almost identical to ... [that] ... found in men' (Verkaik, 1995). They are not alone, however, and this same point is echoed by lobby groups which claim to represent lay interests. The UK Men's Health Forum, founded in 1994 to 'improve the health of men of all ages', has stated that it 'wants to see the subject of male depression discussed at ante-natal classes so that men know what they are suffering from if they develop the condition' (BBC News Online,1999a). Fathers Direct (now known as the Fatherhood Institute), a charity founded in 1999 to promote fathers' involvement with their children, states that 'Fathers' own depression is ... a cause for concern, not least because of its potential to exacerbate maternal depression' (Fathers Direct, 2007), and has argued that more should be done to prevent this problem (BBC News Online, 1999a).

Male PND has also been amplified as a social concern as it has featured regularly over the past decade as the subject matter of newspaper feature articles and opinion pieces about the experience of the contemporary father (Cook, 1995; Johnson, 2003; Lusher & Welsh, 2003). My analysis of 98 newspaper articles about male PND (identified by a search of the British media using the comprehensive on-line media database Lexis Nexis) from 1992, the year that the first newspaper article about this subject appeared in the British press, to 2004, shows almost all journalism has aimed to draw attention to a new and valid problem: most media coverage has endorsed the idea that fathers, just like many mothers, may find parenthood a depressing ordeal. Typical article headlines include, 'The Fathers Who Suffer "Post-Natal Depression"' (Sheppard, 1992), 'The Cradle of Men's Misery' (Marles, 1994) and 'Post-natal Depression Hits New Dads Too' (Peterkin, 2000), with arguments made for recognition of 'the alarming rise in male postnatal depression' (Rawles, 2004).

The idea that it is *helpful* for some men to understand their experience of contemporary fatherhood in an illness framework has dominated public accounts of the subject. The lack of contest over this approach points to an important socio-cultural development. It contrasts strikingly with examples from the past, where attempts to define experience as illness have met with considerable resistance (as was indeed the case for so-called 'female maladies') (Lee & Frayn, 2008). Advocacy for recognition of male PND by a variety of social actors suggests that the representation of fathers' contemporary experience as illness 'makes sense' in contemporary culture. In particular, it suggests that the *emotional life* of the father has emerged as an area of interest and concern. This indicates that the emergence of male PND may be best illuminated through placing it in the context of larger socio-cultural developments, associated with the problematisation of 'male emotions'.

THE CHANGING CONSTRUCTION OF FATHERHOOD

The father identified as 'normal' or 'unproblematic' tends to be absent or largely ignored ... men are positioned as requiring much in the way of expert help in terms of preparing themselves for fatherhood, getting through pregnancy and birth unscathed. Fatherhood is represented as replete with traps for the unprepared and unwary, a profoundly difficult and demanding and potentially emotionally disturbing experience and even a health risk.

(Lupton & Barclay, 1997: 50)

Fatherhood has become the subject of extensive popular, scholarly and official discussion in Britain, and emphasis is often placed on how much fatherhood has changed in recent years (Lewis & O'Brien, 1987; Burghes *et al.*, 1997; Berkmann, 2004; Giles, 2004). Key changes referred to include the shift from fathers never attending the birth of their child to them being almost always present, and growing levels of paternal activity in regard to responsibility for child rearing. Change to fatherhood is widely presented as underpinned by developments in women's social role, in particular to increased female participation in the labour force. Burghes *et al.* (1997) argue in this vein that, as a result of women's changed position in regard to work outside the home, 'Fathers and mothers are expected to share breadwinning with caring for their children and doing the domestic chores, even if attitudes vary about how parents should divide these tasks between them' (1997: 75). Bringing up children has thus come to be increasingly viewed as a male, as much as a female, activity.

However, analyses of representations of social change suggest that the father is often constructed in a way as to draw attention to *his problems* regarding these changes. As the extract above indicates, Lupton and Barclay, on the basis of their review of psychological, family health and welfare, and sociological literature, found that the image of the 'normal' or 'unproblematic' was hard to find. Rather, fatherhood most often represented a risky and dangerous enterprise that men are ill-equipped to confront. As they also note, it is striking that it is both where fathers participate in caring for their children, and where they do not, that men are represented as in some way deficient. Hence both the 'absent father' and the 'new father' are the subjects of worried commentaries.

This concern about fathers and fathering is not entirely new. A common thread of contemporary media, academic and political discourse is the idea of 'masculinity in crisis' (Scourfield & Drakeford, 2002), but the perceived problem of 'crisis' is not restricted to the present. According to historians of the family, in the early decades of the twentieth century anxieties and concerns were expressed in expert and popular literature about the level of involvement of fathers in child rearing, considered problematic because of social and economic changes. They identified 'a transitional process for fathers, or even a "crisis" of masculinity in relation to fatherhood caused by industrialization, the apparent spread and domination of materialist and individualist values' (Lupton & Barclay, 1997: 40–1).

In the late twentieth and early twenty-first century, some new themes are identifiable in the overall discourse of 'crisis', however, and these have drawn especially upon the idea of 'masculinity', usually defined as a set of traits and characteristics. Father-absence is deemed problematic in this vein, since it is considered by many opinion formers necessary for children – male children in particular – to be exposed to 'masculinity' in order for them to develop in an emotionally healthy fashion. Father-presence also becomes a source of concern, however, since involved fatherhood is considered to exist in a tense relationship with 'masculinity'. Thus, note Lupton and Barclay, most literature about the 'involved father' 'tends to represent fatherhood as a potentially pathological experience, replete with upheavals and the need for major adjustments. Such terms as "stress", "strain", "role transition" and "psychological disruption" are frequently used' (1997: 48). It appears in this way that dominant in discussions of what fathers do is a strong tendency to individualise problems by relating fathers' attitudes and practices to male psychology and to draw upon a version of male psychology in which emphasis is placed on its problematic nature of 'male emotions'.

For example, Clive Ballard, a psychiatrist from Birmingham, in his account of why men now suffer from PND, has posed the cause of male PND this way: 'In Britain in the 1950s ... roles were clear-cut. The father went out, earned the salary, came back, had a token play with the baby, and that was the end of it. Now it's not clear what is expected' (Verkaik, 1995). Fatherhood is thus viewed nostalgically, as previously straightforward but presently much more problematic. The explanation for fathers' current experience is their difficulty adapting psychologically to a context where what is expected of them is not as 'clear-cut' as in the 1950s. Echoing this approach, it has been argued that even if they do manage to adapt before fatherhood, having a child brings about a new set of problems. 'New Man', it is argued, has become 'distant and confused New Dad', with fatherhood viewed as the cause of 'a mild form of depression for the modern-day man' (Hill, 2004: 9). In these accounts, male PND clearly has no biological component; its origin lies in the difficulties men are having in responding psychologically to a new and uncertain social context. In this representation of the contemporary father, he tends to appear as a person hampered by 'masculinity' and so unable to change as society changes, because he has to struggle hard with a psychology which has only one emotional 'setting'.

For the purposes of this chapter, however, it is not only the construction of men as emotionally disoriented in the face of new social conditions that is important. The emergence of male PND points to a second dimension regarding claims about the effects of social change for men; this experience of disorientation is *pathologised*. Not simply are men deemed confused and unclear about their social role. Rather they are represented as *made sick* as a result of this confusion. In this light, Furedi's (2004) claim that the process that is most marked currently may be better termed 'psychologization' than 'medicalization' appears insightful. It is experiences, he argues, that involve *emotional processes* that are now especially prone to be described in medical terms. The psychologisation of emotional life takes place as claims-makers, often those who have no association with medicine in a formal sense, 'exporting the ideas of illness and disease beyond the body to make sense of conditions and experiences that are distinctly cultural and social' (Furedi, 2004: 100). According to this account people have, consequently, come to be represented as 'ill' by merit of the effects of their everyday life experiences (experiences which inevitably engage the emotions).

This is an assessment that appears to resonate with the construction of fathers' experience of PND. For example, ambivalence, boredom, frustration and anger, feelings all reported by fathers (and mothers) of their experience, are represented as aspects of male PND (Johnson, 2003; Parkes, 2003; Daniel, 2004; Rawles, 2004). This trend parallels the way that almost any negative experience reported by women about motherhood is now deemed a symptom of 'postnatal illness' leading to the expansive pathologising of maternal experience; it is for this reason that it can now be claimed by some that the vast majority of mothers – 80 per cent according to some accounts – suffer mental illness (Lee, 2003, 2006). The easy incorporation of the experience of challenging emotional experience into a diagnostic framework gives PND the clear hallmark of medicalisation, and in line with medicalisation processes more widely, the solution to the problems is inevitably some form of professional intervention.

The professional management of fatherhood does indeed form a central part of its contemporary construction. As Lupton and Barclay explain, 'the difficulties of fatherhood often tend to be represented ... as individualistic problems that require individual solutions, often assisted by the appropriate "experts"' (Lupton & Barclay 1997: 49). Burghes et al. (1997) point out that, of many initiatives directed at fathers 'A key emphasis today is on increasing the nurturing role of fatherhood' (1997: 88; emphasis added). In other words, men, it is assumed, will find it difficult to be able to take on a role that requires them to form emotionally meaningful relationships with their children, unless action is taken by professionals to enable them to understand how to behave, and a plethora of schemes directed at fathers have emerged as a result (Hume, 2003). The pathologising and professional control of fatherhood also conforms to wider developments in representation of 'male emotions', as I now discuss.

PATHOLOGISING 'MALE EMOTIONS'

Men often bottle things up and live with their problems longer than they need to. This can sometimes lead to stress-related illness ... A lot of men know more about how a car works then their own emotions.

(*Ron Bracey, clinical psychologist, cited in Jackson, 2004*)

Most men don't like to admit that they feel fragile or vulnerable, and so are less likely to talk about their feelings with their friends, loved ones or their doctors. This may be the reason that they often don't ask for help when they become depressed.

(*Royal College of Psychiatrists, 2007*)

Characteristic of contemporary culture is a powerful tendency to represent emotional experience as illness, demonstrated by the ubiquity of terms like stress, addiction, and trauma in descriptions of everyday experience (Peele, 1995; Lee, 2003). The connection has been identified elsewhere between this sort of representation of experience and cultural presumptions about peoples' (in)ability to cope with their emotions. The key point of the diagnosis of experience as illness – for example through the rise of diagnosis of social phobia and anxiety disorder – is the assumption that psychologically, 'individuals lack the resilience to deal with feelings of isolation, disappointment or failure' (Furedi, 2004: 159). Similarly, Summerfield (2001) argues that, with reference to the rapid growth in diagnosis of post-traumatic stress disorder (PTSD), the medicalisation process can be understood as the product of a particular construction of 'personhood' in which it is deemed usual, not rare, for people to be overwhelmed and engulfed by adverse or challenging life events, and thus made ill by their social experience.

What is marked about the present situation, according to these analyses, is the popularity of a view of people that elevates vulnerability and a sense of feeling of being unable to cope with social interactions. It is this which lies behind the expansion of 'mental illness' and, in turn, the widespread advocacy of the need for therapeutic intervention as part of everyday life (Fitzpatrick, 2001). The connection made between an ability to cope with negative or unexpected feelings and illness is at the centre of representations of the cause of wide range of specifically *male* illness. Lupton and Barclay note in the literature on fatherhood that there is a 'focus on the need to counsel men, to allow them to express their feelings ... [which is] typical of the contemporary importance placed in self-expression and therapeutic practice' (1997: 50). The assumption of vulnerability in men is articulated in a particular way, however. What is frequently put forward is the idea that *men are reluctant to admit to vulnerability*, although vulnerability is their authentic state of being. Ron Bracey, quoted above, thus describes men 'bottling things up', and becoming ill as a result. An invitation to admit vulnerability is offered as the solution: as the Royal College of Psychiatrists puts it, an inability to admit feeling fragile is common among men, and it is this inability that fosters depression as man fail to 'seek help'. Encouraging 'help-seeking' becomes in this way the therapeutic imperative to address men's ill health.

The concept of 'masculinity' is central to this therapeutic impulse. Thus, 'Masculinity is among the more significant risk factors associated with men's illness' (Kimmel, 1995: vii). Social psychologists Lee and Owens centre their analysis on 'hegemonic masculinity', defined as 'toughness, unemotionality, physical competence, competitiveness and aggression' (2002: 3). Drawing on terminology developed by Connell (1995), illness-inducing behaviours associated with 'hegemonic masculinity', they claim, include 'relative reluctance to seek help for medical and psychological problems', 'avoidance of the expression of emotion', and 'high-level involvement in risky behaviours, which include both the socially sanctioned risks involved in dangerous sports, and the more deviant masculine-typed risks such as crime and violent behaviour' (2002: 4). As Rosenfeld and Faircloth (2006) note, the dominant trend evident in almost all representation of men's health is, in this way, to 'pathologize masculinity as a health risk and thus take an active role in the contraction of risk society' (2006: 14).

In this framework, the attainment of health is coterminous with encouraging men to adopt a different mindset – crucially one that involves an acceptance of vulnerability, and which embraces the need for 'help'. This mainstream status of this approach is indicated by extent to which the claim that men need to be less 'tough' and 'invulnerable', more 'open' and more prepared to 'seek help' informs British health-related institutions. Official health-promotion programmes in Britain increasingly explicitly target men: New Labour has aimed from the outset to develop 'new schemes to encourage men to be diagnosed earlier and to ensure that health campaigns are aimed at men as well as women'

(Department of Health, 2000). Key organisations including the Royal College of Nursing, the British Medical Association and the Department of Health have presented initiatives that aim to encourage men to 'seek help'. The definition of the problem of male emotions found in claims made about male PND conforms to this approach.

Indeed, health services in some parts of Britain have established initiatives to treat men with PND. In 1995, it was reported that 'Health visitors in North Staffordshire were the first in the country to be specially trained to identify fathers who might be suffering from depression' (Verkaik, 1995). In 2004, this problem was deemed sufficiently extensive to warrant the health service in Basildon, Essex to fund a new scheme called 'Fathers Matter, In Tune With Dads' that offers counselling to men with PND (BBC News Online 2003a, c; McDougall, 2004; Wright, 2004). A spokesman for West Ham United Football Club, sponsors of Fathers Matter, argues that it is ultimately 'macho culture' that is to blame for the problems of fathers: 'Too many young men, who are overjoyed about being a father, can also experience worry and anxiety, which can develop into depression and desperation. There's nothing macho about suffering in silence' (South Essex Partnership NHS Trust, 2004). According to Mary Alabaster, the director of Fathers Matter, the problem is 'traditionally perceived male characteristics such as being physically and emotionally strong and self-contained [since they] impede the ability to either ask for help or show vulnerability' (Daniel, 2004: 209).

Help-seeking behaviour is valorised through such claims, and attempts to 'cope alone' without professional support are stigmatised. In discussion of male PND, one form the validation of professional intervention takes is in the definition of men as 'excluded', and needing to be, in contrast, 'included'. As Mary Alabaster explains it, 'Let us include dads and advocate for this group in society … We need to tune in to fathers and can start that by addressing their psychological needs – that means *not* excluding them … and treating them as an inconvenience' (Daniel, 2004: 208). Curham (2000), author of an advice book on PND, makes similar claims in her representation of fathers, arguing that men are 'forgotten victims' in regard to PND. While they can find themselves 'quite depressed' after the birth of a child, unlike women, they have nowhere to go to find help. 'Becoming a father can have a huge impact on a man and yet all the attention seems to be focused on the woman' (2000: 72).

To this end of 'inclusion', Fathers Matter has developed its own 'screening tool', a series of questions asked of new parents to identify those 'at risk' from PND, notably entitled the Vulnerability Index, to be used by midwives and health visitors during the women's pregnancy. Questions asked by those using the scale concern 'awareness of possible changes that can occur in a relationship during the antenatal or postnatal period', with lack of 'awareness' indicating 'vulnerability'. Participants are also asked, 'Do you drink alcohol?' and 'Do you use any street or non-prescribed drugs?' Like the more frequently used scale to measure female PND, the Edinburgh Postnatal Depression Scale (EPDS), these questions are broad and vague, and are thus liable to generate a large number of women and men considered 'at risk' of suffering from PND (Lee, 2003). Those it 'includes' on this basis are also subject to a particular construction of the problems they face. They are not of an economic or social type; they are of a psychological order. They are not 'excluded' by merit of their social or economic position, but because their feelings have not been recognised by professionals. The professional management of their transition to fatherhood becomes the solution advocated to the problems of fathers today.

CONCLUSION

In Britain, in the course of about 15 years, male PND has become a visible social problem. As I described at the outset, it has been the subject of discussion that has largely presented male PND as a valid health problem deserving of recognition. It has been argued that a range of claimsmakers have played a part in this particular construction of male PND, including some psychiatrists, other health professionals, and campaign groups. It is in this context that male PND can be seen as an example of a wider development, in which ideas about illness have been exported beyond the physical body and applied to a social and personal experience; although men do not become pregnant and give birth, they have nevertheless been constructed as suffering from PND as a result of their fatherhood role. Through this process of export, it is the social state of fatherhood that has been medicalised and, concomitantly, it has come to be viewed as connected with the development of illness.

In sociological terms, the application of medical labels to the experience of both sexes through the expansion of the category PND can perhaps best be conceptualised as a reflection of a two-sided development. On the one hand, men and women are now increasingly deemed equal within the family and in society more broadly. In Britain, however, they are also deemed more equal in relation to the difficulties they are considered likely to encounter when attempting to cope emotionally as parents. One conclusion that can be drawn is that in contemporary culture women and men are constructed as at once more equal, but at the same time both more vulnerable and helpless than in the past. Where once the majority of parents were expected to be able to respond adequately to the demands of parenthood, the notion of vulnerability has expanded to the point where the inability to cope as a parent has been normalised. This process of expansion has meant that not only are the psychological demands of the motherhood role frequently considered so overwhelming that most mothers are deemed to suffer depression – the expectation that fatherhood in its contemporary form is also too psychologically demanding for many men to cope with has also gained a great deal of ground.

The merits of this construction of men and women as commonly vulnerable need to be debated. Those who advocate recognition of male PND and the consequent provision of 'support' represent this as an act that can 'empower' men, women and children. The attribution of illness status is thus represented as a very positive step. An alterative account would contend that it might, in contrast, have the result of intensifying, rather than diminishing, the feelings of powerlessness and confusion that advocates of this diagnosis claim they seek to alleviate through giving fathers' experience a medical label. Given that advocacy of recognition of illness on the grounds that it empowers is now commonplace, further research and discussion about the implications of this development is an important task to undertake.

REFERENCES

American Psychiatric Association (2001) Factsheet: Postpartum Depression. Washington, DC: American Psychiatric Association, July.

Ballard, C.G., Davis, R., Cullen, P.C., Mohan, R.N. & Dean, C. (1994) Prevalence of postnatal psychiatric morbidity in mothers and fathers. *British Journal of Psychiatry*, 164: 782–8.

BBC News Online (1999a) Men suffer from baby blues. http://news.bbc.co.uk, 4 May.

BBC News Online (1999b) New fathers get advice. http://news.bbc.co.uk, 10 September.

BBC News Online (2003a) Advice for baby blues dads. http://news.bbc.co.uk, 24 August.

BBC News Online (2003b) Anorexia 'overlooked in boys'. http://news.bbc.co.uk, 29 August.

BBC News Online (2003c) New advice service for fathers. http://news.bbc.co.uk, 27 December.

BBC News Online (2004) Self-harm 'growing issue for men'. http://news.bbc.co.uk, 28 July.

Berkmann, M. (2004) *Fatherhood: The Truth*. London: Vermilion.

Brockington, I. (1996) *Motherhood and Mental Illness*. Oxford: Oxford University Press.

Burghes, L., Clarke, L. & Cronin, N. (1997) *Fathers and Fatherhood in Britain*. London: Family Policy Studies Centre.

Coltman, N. (1998) Baby blues hits dads too. *Newcastle Evening Chronicle*, 26 November.

Connell, R.W. (1995) *Masculinities*. Cambridge: Polity.

Conrad, P. (1992) Medicalization and social control. *Annual Review of Sociology*, 18: 209–32.

Conrad, P. & Potter, D. (2000) From hyperactive children to ADHD adults: observations on the expansion of medical categories. *Social Problems*, 47(4): 559–82.

Cook, E. (1995) Tears before bedtime – from dad. *The Independent*, 1 February.

Curham, S. (2000) *Antenatal and Postnatal Depression, Practical Advice and Support for All Sufferers*. London: Vermilion.

Dalton, K. and Holton, W.M. (2001) *Depression after Childbirth*. Oxford: Oxford University Press.

Daniel, K. (2004) Fathers' psychological needs – a neglected area. *Community Practitioner*, 77(6): 208–9.

Department of Health. (2000) Health Minister to announce new plans to improve men's health. Press release, http://www.dh.gov.uk/en/Publicationsandstatistics/Pressreleases/DH_4002600), accessed 28 January 2008.

Ehrenreich, B. and English, D. (1973) *Complaints and Disorders: The Sexual Politics of Sickness*. New York: Feminist Press.

Fathers Direct. (2007) Fathers and post-natal depression. www.fathersdirect.com, accessed 12 December 2007.

Figert, A. E. (1996) *Women and the Ownership of PMS: The Structuring of a Psychiatric Disorder*. New York: Aldine de Gruyter.

Figes, K. (1998) *Life after Birth*. London: Penguin.

Fitzpatrick, M. (2001) *The Tyranny of Health, Doctors and the Regulation of Lifestyle*. London and New York: Routledge.

Furedi, F. (2004). *Therapy Culture: Cultivating Vulnerability in and Uncertain Age*. London: Routledge.

Furedi, F. (2006) The end of professional dominance. *Society*, 43(6): 14–18.

Furedi, F. (2008) Medicalization in therapy culture. In D. Wainwright (ed.), *A Sociology of Health*. London: Sage.

Giles, S. (2004) *From Lad to Dad: How to Survive as a Pregnant Father*. London: White Ladder Press.

Goodman, J.H. (2004) Paternal postpartum depression, its relationship to maternal postpartum depression, and implications for family health. *Journal of Advanced Nursing*, 45(1): 26–35.

Hardyment, C. (2002) *Perfect Parents*. Oxford and New York: Oxford University Press.

Hill, R. (2004) How New Man turned into distant, confused New Dad. *Observer*, 20 June.

Huang, C.C. & Warner, L.A. (2005) Relationship characteristics and depression and fathers with newborns. *Social Service Review*, 79: 95–118.

Hume, M. (2003) How did we fathers manage before 'Dad' told us not to drop the baby on its head? *The Times*, 9 April.

Jackson, M. (2004) Men are not too macho to cry. http://news.bbc.co.uk, 4 July.

Johnson, P. (2003) The baby blues nearly killed me. *Mirror*, 23 August.

Kimmel, M. S. (1995) Series editor's introduction. In D. Sabo & D.F. Gordon (eds), *Men's Health and Illness*. London: Sage, pp. vii–viii.

Kukla, R. (2005) *Mass Hysteria, Medicine, Culture and Women's Bodies*. New York, Rowman & Littlefield.

Lee, E. (2003) *Abortion, Motherhood and Mental Health: Medicalizing Reproduction in the United States and Great Britain*. New York: Aldine de Gruyter.

Lee, E. (2006) Medicalizing motherhood. *Society*, 43(6): 47–50.

Lee, E. & Frayn, L. (2008) The feminization of health. In D. Wainwright (ed.), *A Sociology of Health*. London: Sage.

Lee, C. & Owens, R.G. (2002) *The Psychology of Men's Health*. Buckingham and Philadelphia: Open University Press.

Lewis, C. & O'Brien, M. (1987) *Reassessing Fatherhood: New Observations on Fathers and the Modern Family*. London: Sage.

Lupton, D. & Barclay, L. (1997) *Constructing Fatherhood: Discourses and Experiences*. London: Sage.

Lusher, A. & Welsh, B. (2003) Men to get counselling for 'postnatal depression'. *Sunday Telegraph*, 24 August.

Marles, K. (1994) The cradle of men's misery. *Independent* (Sunday Review), 20 March.

Matthey, S., Barnett, B.E., Kavanagh, D.J. & Howie, P. (2001) Validation of the Edinburgh Postnatal Depression Scale for men, and comparison of item endorsement with the partners. *Journal of Affective Disorders*, 64: 175–84.

McDougall, L. (2004) Fathers urged to admit that they get the baby blues too. *Sunday Herald*, 14 March.

Miles, A. (1991) *Women, Health and Medicine*. Milton Keynes and Philadelphia: Open University Press.

Nicolson, P. (2000) Competing explanations of postpartum depression: what are the benefits to women? In J. Ussher (ed.), *Women's Health: Contemporary International Perspectives*. Leicester: BPS Books.

Oakley, A. (1980) *Women Confined: Towards a New Sociology of Childbirth*. Oxford: Martin Robertson.

Orvice, V. (1994) The new man gets the baby blues. *Daily Mail*, 23 June.

Parkes, D. (2003) Support for men with baby blues. *Birmingham Evening Mail*, 22 October.

Peele, S. (1995) *Diseasing of America: How We Allowed Recovery Zealots and the Treatment Industry to Convince Us We Are Out of Control*. San Francisco: Jossey-Bass.

Peterkin, T. (2000) Post-natal depression hits new dads too. *Scotland on Sunday*, 17 September.

Rawles, S. (2004) Birthing pains. *Observer Magazine*, 21 March. http://observer.guardian.co.uk/magazine/story/0,,1172622,00.html, accessed 28 January 2008.

Riessman, C. K. (1983) Women and medicalization: a new perspective. *Social Policy*, Summer: 3–17.

Rosenfeld, D. & Faircloth, C. (2006) Introduction. In Rosenfeld & Faircloth (eds), *Medicalized Masculinities*. Philadelphia: Temple University Press, pp. 1–20.

Royal College of Psychiatrists (2007) Men and depression. www.rcpsych.ac.uk.

Scourfield, J. & Drakeford, M. (2002) New Labour and the 'problem of men'. *Critical Social Policy*, 22(4): 619–40.

Sheppard, F. (1992) The fathers who suffer 'post-natal depression'. *Daily Mail*, 14 September.

Sheringham, S. (2003) Men to get NHS counselling for postnatal depression. *PA News*, 23 August.

South Essex Partnership NHS Trust (2004) Fathers matter. Press release, 28 January. www.southessex-trust.nhs.uk.

Summerfield, D. (2001) The invention of post-traumatic stress disorder and the social usefulness of a psychiatric category. *British Medical Journal*, 322: 95–8.

Tavris, C. (1992) *The Mismeasure of Woman*. New York: Simon & Schuster.

Verkaik, R. (1995) Men with the baby blues. *Sunday Times*, 31 December.

Welford, H. (2002) *Feelings after Birth*. London: National Childbirth Trust.

Wolf, N. (2001) *Misconceptions, Truth, Lies and the Unexpected on the Journey to Motherhood*. London: Chatto & Windus..

Wright, O. (2004) Fathers at risk of postnatal depression as well. *The Times*, 20 March.

10 PROSTATE CANCER AND MASCULINITIES IN AUSTRALIA

Alex Broom

INTRODUCTION

Prostate cancer is an increasingly high-profile issue in contemporary Australian society, and for sociologists, it represents a key site of interplay between cultural practices around masculinity and men's health and well-being. Australian sensibilities around masculinity have received considerable attention from scholars in recent years (Connell, 2000, 2005) and the enactment of cultural ideals around manliness have been linked to a wide range of health issues, including prostate cancer (e.g. Oliffe, 2005, 2006). Contemporary masculinities, in their various forms, are increasingly cited as interacting problematically with key elements of prostate cancer care (e.g. Chapple & Ziebland, 2002), including testing, treatment and post-treatment side effects. Indeed, each stage in the disease and treatment process *potentially* presents quite specific challenges to many men's sense of masculine identity (as defined through control, strength and agility) and their ability to perform core elements of their identity work (for example, potency and continence). Despite increasing recognition of this problematic of identity disruption amongst Australian men who have experienced prostatic disease (Broom, 2004, 2005; Oliffe, 2004, 2005, 2006), little research has been done in the area.

As seen internationally, there is a paucity of academic research, community support and public awareness in and around prostate cancer. Significantly, *all* forms of social support and state funding for prostate cancer in Australia lag behind those associated with breast cancer, with which, considering its prevalence and gender-specificity, one might make a comparison (Broom, 2004; PCFA, 2008). In many ways prostate cancer reflects a broader rather than a specific site of cultural avoidance and denial in relation to men's health and well-being (Connell, 2005). The notion of the archetypal 'Aussie male' is centred on such things as beer-drinking, barbecues and sport, with talking about emotions or help-seeking high on the cultural list of 'things to avoid'. As such, Australian men have higher mortality rates than women for all major causes of death and their use of health services is 40 per cent lower than that of Australian women, even taking into account childbirth (Broom, 2004). Moreover, whilst the deeply embodied and highly traumatising nature of biomedical oncological interventions for breast cancer patients is regularly discussed in the public sphere (e.g. art exhibitions) and in public forums by high-profile individuals (e.g. the impact of mastectomy on feminine identity), the cultural silences around the implications of prostate cancer for Australian men are, by comparison, deafening. This is particularly concerning given the strength of masculine ideals in the Australian cultural landscape and the potential for them to further problematise help-seeking for, and experiences of, prostatic disease.

As such, the study discussed in this chapter sought to examine, for the first time, the complex intersectionality in Australia between men's gender identities and experiences of prostate cancer pre-, peri- and post-treatment. What emerged was a patterned complexity in their accounts of disease and treatment processes, with each, albeit differentially, experiencing prostate cancer as a significant challenge for their senses of self and masculinity. Moreover, it would seem that the lived experiences of decision-making and biomedical interventions are inextricably tied to the enactment of cultural codes of masculinity.

PROSTATE CANCER AND CONTEMPORARY MASCULINITIES

Rates of prostate cancer in Australia are high and on the increase, with around one in nine men in Australia developing prostate cancer in their lifetime (PCFA, 2008). Prostate cancer is the most common cancer diagnosis in Australian males, and the second most common cause of death. Men are living longer, giving prostatic malignancies more time to spread beyond the prostate with potentially fatal consequences. The erstwhile maxim, 'men die with it not of it', is certainly not true today. Younger men are now developing prostate cancer, and many die of the disease and not with it (Frydenberg, 1998; Broom, 2004). The number of new cases of prostate cancer in Australia increased by 12.7 per cent from 12,003 in 2002 to 13,526 in 2003, overtaking colorectal cancer as Australia's most common cancer (excluding non-melanocytic skin cancer). The next most common cancers are breast cancer, melanoma of the skin and lung cancer (AIHW, 2007). Every year around 3,000 Australian men die of prostate cancer.

The result of this trend is that there are *much* larger numbers of Australian men opting for at least one (and sometimes more than one) of the major treatment options available for prostate cancer, introducing a range of problematic side effects and quality-of-life issues. The main treatment options currently include surgery (e.g. radical prostatectomy, involving removal of the prostate), radiation treatment (e.g. brachytherapy, involving targeted radiation), hormone therapy and watchful waiting. As a result of the aforementioned increases in morbidity, hospital admissions for a principal diagnosis of prostate cancer almost doubled from 13,715 in 2000–01 to 25,429 in 2005–06 (AIHW, 2007) and radical prostatectomies increased by 56 per cent in the same period, from 6,088 to 9,478. Radical prostatectomy represents a very serious and potentially life-threatening operation, with serious side effects even from successful surgery, including pain, incontinence and impotence (Oliffe, 2005). Whilst trying to reduce mortality has been a major focus in the biomedical literature (e.g. Lu-Yao *et al.*, 2002), it is argued here that a focus on the lived experiences of men pre-, peri- and post treatment remains critical in terms of better understanding and dealing with the psychosocial impacts of prostate cancer.

There has been some work done internationally on various facets of men's experiences of prostate cancer. In terms of the limitations of existing clinical contexts for dealing with men's emotional and psychosocial issues, a recent study by Korfage *et al.* (2006) found that existing quality-of-life measures tend to create the illusion that men are *not* concerned about the impacts of surgery, concealing issues around impotency and incontinence. Sociological work in the area, however, has vividly illustrated the impact of prostatic intervention on men's senses of identity and overall well-being. In their examination of the interplay of masculinity and prostatic disease, Chapple & Ziebland (2002) explored the ways in which various side effects of prostate cancer reduced some men's senses of masculinity and argued for a focus on *both* physicality and cultural practice when exploring how illness may affect men. Oliffe (2006) explored this intersectionality of culture and physicality in his Australian research, examining the relationships between masculine identity and experiences of androgen deprivation therapy (hormone therapy), and found that such interventions affect men in deeply gendered ways, impacting on their relationships and identities. He also explored men's experiences of radical prostatectomies and the ways in which they go about redefining their sexuality and masculinity following surgically induced impotence (Oliffe, 2005). Despite this emerging work in the area, there is still little awareness of, or research into, the effects of prostate cancer treatments on Australian masculinities. By contrast, the effect of surgical techniques (mastectomy versus lumpectomy) on femininity has been thoroughly investigated (e.g. Langellier & Sullivan, 1998; Broom, 2001; Kiss & Meryn, 2001).

Theoretically, of interest here is the intersectionality between culture, disease and biomedical technologies. In particular, the ways in which particular cultural practices around masculinity are 'done' or 'accomplished' (Connell, 2005) and how prostate cancer and biomedical interventions contribute to an 'undoing' (or require a reconstruction of) some men's senses of self and identity. It should be emphasised that multiplicity within such experiences is also key as it is increasingly recognised that masculinity is a highly differentiated and indeed temporal cultural practice (Courtenay, 2000; Connell, 2005). Initial work in the area of men's health tended to reify simplistic and overly linear conceptions of hegemonic masculinity (and its interplay with poor health outcomes), whereas more recently work has focused on the highly differentiated grass-roots experiences of masculine identity and selfhood (e.g. Chapple & Ziebland, 2002; Oliffe, 2005, 2006; Robertson, 2006). Specifically, how sexuality, ethnicity, geography, age and other biographical factors mediate the enactment of masculinity and thus men's experiences of illness and disease. As such, masculinity is here viewed as multiple and temporal, and as reconstructable and malleable both in terms of wider cultural practice and individual conceptions of the self and identity.

Hitherto there has been little work examining the relationship between masculinities and prostate cancer. As such, the study reported on here begins to fill this void, qualitatively exploring a group of men's experiences of being tested, investigated and treated for prostate cancer. In doing so it provides much needed insight, illustrating that, at least for the men in this study, masculinity prevails as a central concern within the treatment of prostate cancer, often superseding the threat of mortality, and thus fundamentally shaping their treatment decisions.

METHOD

In total, 33 men were recruited to participate in the study. Interviews continued until the sample included men with a range of prognoses, who had been through a range of treatments. All the men were interviewed in their own homes for 1–2 hours. Although generally following the principles of in-depth interviewing outlined by such authors as Rice and Ezzy (1999) and Minichiello (1995), a flexible approach was taken, adapting, as seemed appropriate in each interview, to the particular respondent. Resistance to seeking help and advice, negative experiences of biomedical procedures, and the difficulties posed by treatment side effects each emerged as important themes in the interviews and are central to the following discussion. Drawn primarily from prostate cancer support groups, the sample probably represents a more educated group, less dominated by traditional ideas of masculinity than the larger population of older men with prostate cancer. Further research is needed, but it may be that the concerns raised by these men are amplified within the wider population of men suffering from prostatic disease.

CULTURES OF MASCULINITY AND THEIR IMPACT ON HEALTH

Before we examine the intersections of biomedical intervention and identity in the context of prostate cancer, it is useful to examine these men's narratives around the broader cultural practices and understandings around masculinity. In order to critically examine men's experiences of vulnerability in the clinical environment or their resistance to transrectal procedures, it is useful to first consider wider socio-cultural beliefs and processes about 'men' (and Australian men in particular) which provide a platform for these experiences. The interviews were conducted in such a way that, to provide a context, dialogue began as a series of interactional reflections of Australian masculinities and their impact of men's health. As a result, the interviews provided considerable insight into men's views of and approaches to health and illness and their relationship to idealised forms of masculinity. In particular, cultural stereotypes and educational processes (both formal and informal) were viewed as crucial in shaping men's views of their health and their bodies, and importantly, their help-seeking. In the following excerpts, two respondents talk about 'being men', masculinity and their relationship to health behaviour:

Interviewee: Men don't want to get their health checked.
Interviewer: Why do you think that is?
Interviewee: I think it's part of the male image thing, part of the cultural thing ... that the male role was to be the strong healthy person who was the breadwinner, all of that sort of stuff. That's gradually changing, whereas the women were meant to be the ones who got ill and had all these problems. So there's that cultural thing. I think it's changing but there's also; well, men aren't supposed to get ill. It's a macho thing. Women have been educated to go and get checked up routinely, men haven't been. Every girl is now educated that you go and get a pap smear. That means every two years a female goes to see a doctor and as soon as they walk in the door if they are a good doctor, they are observing other things apart from the fact that you're wanting a pap smear. We have no similar system with males that sort of says, well, every couple of years you go and see a doctor. (6 months post-treatment, organ-confined disease, 40–50 years)

Another respondent comments:

This sort of macho thing ... 'I'm not going to let anyone else know I've got the problem and I'm going to figure it out myself ...' [pause] I guess it depends what sort of a wife you've got [laughs]. If you've got a wife who takes some interest in your health you get pushed into it. But for a single guy who has to make these decisions on his own, unless there is something drastically wrong, he's probably not going to do anything. Then you are left with the result of your negligence. You've got to overcome this masculinity thing. (3 years post-treatment, organ-confined disease, 61–70 years)

As shown in the above excerpts and in the interviews with the other men, there emerged a sense of the considerable pressure put on men within the Australian context to 'be well' and 'be strong'. This was in turn linked to their ability to seek help or support for health problems:

> *men tend not to be well-informed about their prostate gland ... they are expected to be well. (1–5 years-post-treatment, organ-confined disease, internet user, 51–60 years)*

Another respondent comments:

> *I had, for years, suffered a slight dribble problem which I was embarrassed about. I didn't realise [sad laugh] prostate cancer was something I should have discussed, because, certainly, I'm not a great socialiser, but even so, the guys I went with, most of them would ... the main topic of conversation would be sport, occasionally politics, mainly sport, and 'How about another drink?' and that was it. (Approx 1 year post-treatment, organ-confined disease, 61–70 years)*

Another respondent comments:

> *It's one of those things that you just don't talk about. You know – men don't talk about prostate – we don't have any problems down there. (1 year post-treatment, organ-confined disease, 61–70 years)*

The cultural construction that 'men aren't supposed to get ill', so evident in these men's accounts, was perceived to be reinforced by the lack of routine structures to assess men's health. Women, it was argued by a number of the men interviewed, are expected to get regular checks for a range of potential health risks. This is not to say that this is necessarily a positive expectation, as one could argue that these cultural expectations contribute to the medicalisation and monitoring of women's bodies. Furthermore, there are considerable problems with the actual effects of monitoring both breast cancer and prostate cancer in terms of the degree to which early diagnosis actually lowers mortality. It is not argued here that women are in a better position through a cultural expectation that they should be 'healthy' and 'aware of risks'; rather, that the set of expectations facing men have particular consequences which hitherto have been given little attention.

One of the respondents talked about how he felt when he first found out he had prostate cancer in relation to cultural expectations and male behaviour:

I had the operation in June and I joined the prostate group in about September. I found it of assistance just to get off my chest the fact that I ... I felt such a goose. Here was a critically important part of my body which I had never come across. I had never ever seen before a diagram showing what the prostate was, what it did, and how critical it was to a very important part of my life. And it's not as if we had any decent sexual education. All they taught us about apart from the amoeba was the frog and the sex act was never even discussed. It was purely coincidental – you didn't know why it dropped its sperm around the eggs – there was never any explanation. But it was infuriating that really ... at school you learnt the basic digestive system, the cardiovascular system, even the rudiments of the nervous system, but the reproduction system was not even mentioned. It would have helped me if the subject matter had been discussed as it has been over the last few years. I would have known that I had a problem. I mean I never had any pains or anything ... I was having difficulty going to the toilet. It's not the sort of thing I would have discussed with another man. And I would have been extremely surprised if another guy had said anything to me about it. Because we tend to be peculiar creatures whereas the ladies have got it all sorted out because of childbirth at a very early age they start talking to each other. They have these sorts of situations. Men don't have problems. Quite a lot of my friends ... some I have lost because of this ... don't go to the doctor – 'I haven't been to the doctor for twenty-five years', they say. (Approximately 1 year post-treatment, organ-confined disease, 61–70 years)

This quote captures a common frustration cited by almost all of the men interviewed here. Until presenting with symptoms, they did not know they had a prostate, what it did. This is significant on a number of different levels. First, the educational context from which many of these men emerged was particularly limited in terms of sexual education or education about men's reproductive systems. As a result, the above respondent's knowledge was nonexistent in terms of the role of the prostate in reproduction. The result is a sense of infuriation of 'not being told' and subsequently feeling 'incredibly foolish'. He had had progressive urination problems for 20 years before he was diagnosed with prostate cancer and never told anyone. In his words, 'I just thought it was a normal part of ageing because no one ever told me any different.' Furthermore, he stated that he would have never told his friends about his problem and would not have expected them to tell him about their health problems.

What emerges is a view of the formal and informal systems that actualise societal constructions of masculinity in terms of their impact on men's approach to health care. The educational system (bearing in mind that for these men this is the Australian educational system of the early to mid-twentieth century) is seen to institutionalise distinctions between men and women in terms of their need for information about their bodies, and cultural norms reflect these institutional practices, whereby men become resistant to talking about their bodies and their health. Each actively contributes to the development of the other; 'maleness' is both institutionally socialised and informally socialised in the process of the ongoing production of the 'male' approach to health. Statements like 'I haven't been to the doctor in twenty-five years' reinforce the 'appropriateness' of denial or complacency, constructing avoidance as a quality to be admired, and the non-examined body as the strong body. This is not to suggest that there is one 'male approach' to health, or that when men talk about 'the male approach', that they are necessarily talking about the same thing. Rather, there are a variety of experiences of, and representations of, 'the male approach' and that these have a significant impact on some of men's experiences of disease.

A testament to the complex and often contradictory views of the impact of masculinity is seen in the accounts of the men who stated that masculinity, as they viewed it, had no particular impact on their disease experience and they considered that 'men who take the macho approach are stupid':

Interviewer: How do you see the treatments for prostate cancer as impacting on men's sense of masculinity?

Interviewee: Boys are brought up not to cry and be very macho and all that sort of thing. It's very hard for me to see where other guys are coming from in that regard. I guess for some men their masculinity is threatened by surgery or something or treatment for prostate cancer.

Interviewer: Do you think it is a big issue?

Interviewee: I think it's an important issue for the guys that it concerns – it's very within that group, but defining that group, I wouldn't have a clue who is thinking along those lines. Certainly my sexual activity has been put on hold. Maybe I'll get that back again, maybe I never will, but I guess as you get older your sexual activity is going to decline to a certain extent anyway. My brother said he is not going to let anyone stick anything up his backside. That's an issue as well for a lot of people. (6 months post initial treatment, organ-confined disease, 61–70 years)

As was the case with several of the respondents, this respondent considered masculinity an important issue and his sexual activity as a significant part of his life, but his sense of 'being a man' was not going to get in the way of seeking information or his treatment decision. His discussion about his brother is significant for the fact that attitudes may in fact change post-diagnosis as men become less focused on particular constructions of masculinity and the stigma of particular tests, focusing more on cure and other facets of their lives that become more important. Although this study does not extend to examining this issue, it would be interesting to examine the importance or implications of masculinity pre-diagnosis and post-diagnosis. Having cancer almost certainly has implications for these men's gender identities in terms of the degree to which they will uphold particular values as important when faced with potentially terminal disease. However, as will be shown in the following sections, the desire to maintain their sense of masculinity may in fact prevail.

Like the previous respondent, and as seen in the following excerpt, several of the other men disputed the importance of masculinity, both in their disease experience, and men's health beliefs and behaviours:

I never felt [masculinity] was a problem for me, but I could certainly imagine that it could be for other men. I used to explain this by the fact that I was a [scientist] and was used to talking a [scientific] approach to things. The much less secure area is that – I think that's an idea which is encouraged by society's propaganda. I've never felt that men were that reluctant to talk about things – this is the idea that this promulgates … I think it is a factor but it's a much more subtle one than the discussion seems to make it. I think you could make up all sorts of reasons if men aren't talking about their health and one of them is that there are less well-documented, well thought-out recommendations for men. This is part of the bigger question of making this information more available. (Mid-treatment, extra-capsular disease, 71–80 years)

This statement outlines a very important point in relation to the issue of masculinity and men's health. To what degree is the so-called 'male approach' a result of a lack of institutional support networks rather than men's desire not to address their health problems? It is argued here that in fact it is a complex combination of these and other factors which are self-perpetuating. For the above respondent, societal or media constructions of the 'male approach' were misrepresentations, constructing males as non-communicative and 'reluctant to talk about things', whereas in his experience this is in fact inaccurate, undermining the 'reality' that many men are very open to talking about their health and sensitive issues such as sexual function and continence. He viewed this as propaganda that 'made men think that they should be like this'. Here he is pointing to the very process by which the representation produces that of which it speaks – the process of producing categories and of generating qualities and attributes of which the media plays a pivotal role. This is the activity of sorting what is 'masculine' from 'feminine', constituting the subject, cementing particular translations of gender; translations which have powerful and important effects on some men and their disease experiences.

Discussion thus far has focused on general perceptions and experiences of being men, with reflection on the implications of cultural understandings of masculinity for health knowledge and help-seeking behaviour. But how do these understandings shape men's experience once they enter the health-care system? How does the need to 'be a man' – to perform certain forms of masculinity – impact on men's experiences of treatment for prostate cancer? What role, if any, do men's gender identities play in decision-making processes?

THE INTERPLAY OF TECHNOLOGY AND IDENTITY IN PROSTATE CANCER CARE

A key line of investigation in the current study was the intersectionality of identity and biomedical procedures and technologies in the realm of prostate cancer care. What were men's experiences of diagnosis, treatment and side effects, and to what degree were these mediated by, or embedded within, cultural discourses and expectations regarding masculinity? As such, within the interviews the men were asked to talk about their experiences of biomedical investigation, diagnosis and treatment. Perhaps unsurprisingly, all the men talked about the broader difficulties posed by these processes (e.g. fear of terminality, pain, anxiety and depression), but also the specific implications for their identities as men. Some of the most striking reflections came in the form of their stories about undergoing particular procedures. The digital rectal examination (DRE), the transrectal ultrasound and the prostate biopsy were a particular focus – a clear similarity being that they are all transrectal procedures. In particular, the prostate biopsy was regularly cited as an experience that intersected with these men's perceptions of 'being men' (see also Oliffe, 2004). The experience of the prostate biopsy was articulated by several of the men with words like 'shame', 'embarrassment' and 'humiliation'. Three respondents reflect on their experiences of the biopsy:

> So I went to the urologists locally here who gave me the usual test with the finger and had a look without doing a biopsy. We talked about it and then they decided a couple of weeks later that they would do biopsies. And that wasn't impressive at all – at your age you probably haven't had one but I think all urologists should have to have a biopsy as part of their training. For most guys it's the most nauseating thing. (1–5 years post-treatment, organ-confined disease, 61–70 years)

Another respondent comments:

> I thought I was going to get a happy needle[1] at least when I had the biopsy done. I'm very sensitive about my genitalia and I think most men are. I'm not blasé about it because it's not the biggest in the world but to go in there … to have the biopsy done I went in and had an enema which was embarrassing enough as it was and then wheeled down to radiology on this trolley and here I am with my bum sticking out the side of the trolley with this stupid little bloody hospital gown on which you might as well not have on …Then, I've got a nurse standing in front of me and I've got two blokes behind me, one obviously manipulating the probe and so forth and the other guy taking the biopsies, he was probably from pathology. I don't think I've been so bloody embarrassed or full of shame. (1–5 years post-treatment, organ-confined disease, 51–60 years)

Another respondent comments:

> I've decided that I'm never having another biopsy if it's not done with a sedative. It's a terrible procedure. It's humiliating, painful and just terrible. Not something anyone should have to go through. It's worse than something being stuck up your old fellow. (Post-treatment, organ-confined disease, 51–60 years)

These excerpts illustrate the effects of procedures like the prostate biopsy can have on men's sense of masculinity and pride (which, for some, are explicitly linked). Feeling exposed, humiliated and, in the first respondent's case, dressed in childlike or feminine attire (i.e. the 'gown' or 'nightie'), several of these men experienced these procedures as problematic for their sense of masculinity and self-respect. A man of well over six feet, and probably weighing in excess of 100 kg, the first respondent shown above was not provided with attire substantial enough to cover his body, undermining his sense of control and strength, and exposing the stereotypical 'measure of masculinity' – the penis. These seemingly mundane procedures such as being wheeled through the hospital or dressed in a 'stupid little hospital gown' – pacification and exposure – all complicated the performance of masculinity for these men.

The impact of transrectal procedures on some of these men's senses of masculinity was significant. As stated by the above respondents, a number of the men reported feeling humiliated when undergoing transrectal procedures, suggesting that, in some way, these procedures compromised their sense of masculinity. It is particularly interesting that this stigma was not mediated by age, with the following two men demonstrating the overall pattern in the interviews and showing that this stigma spans the generations:

> No one likes that idea of it [a rectal examination] and you certainly don't go around talking about it. I didn't tell anyone that I had prostate cancer, I haven't told any of my friends, because they don't understand, you tell people you've got any type of cancer and they think you're dead and buried – it could affect your relationships with people. So my friends and close friends don't know that I have prostate cancer. I was also reluctant to tell any of my family; I've got five children. (1–5 years post-treatment, hormone treatment, extracapsular disease, 71–80 years)

Another respondent comments:

> It's not something that you feel comfortable talking about with other men. There's a bit of stigma associated with rectal [examinations]. (6 months post-treatment, organ-confined disease, 40–50 years)

It was not that these men would not undergo the procedures because of this, but rather, that the procedures had a significant impact on their sense of pride. Although each of the men differed in their level of negativity towards transrectal examinations, they were unanimously negative, and pointed to the 'nature of them' as important. More than the pain, the pre-eminent issue was that the procedures were rectal rather than another entry point. Within the interviews it seemed that it was the very nature of these procedures and the connotations associated with rectal penetration that produced the degree of negativity expressed by the men. Clearly, the classic 'source' of heterosexual masculinity is the penis and male–female intercourse and the majority of the interviewees were married, heterosexual males. This is distinct from penetration of the male rectum, which is generally associated with homoerotic behaviour and very much sits in opposition to dominant forms of heterosexual masculinity. Clearly, transrectal procedures are extremely uncomfortable procedures to undergo and are in no way linked to sexual pleasure. However, there is a clear relationship between these men's senses of how their masculinity may be compromised and the nature of the procedures used in the diagnosis and treatment of prostate cancer (e.g. digital rectal examination, transrectal ultrasound and biopsy). For several of these men, their performances of masculinity (see Butler, 1990) were very much tied to heterosexuality – (see also Gray *et al.*, 2002; Potts, 2000) thus these interventions problematised this by signifying that which runs counter to normative and regulatory (see Foucault, 1977) constructs of masculinity – homoeroticism. Such hegemonic constructions of masculinity as anti-homosexual (as well as anti-feminine) have considerable implications for men in clinical settings. An enduring homophobia within this male population creates an additional layer of complexity within disease and treatment processes, adding to the spectrum of challenges presented by prostate cancer (i.e. the state of being 'ill' and subsequent treatment side effects), further complicating their attempts to retain a 'masculine' identity.

Despite a number of negative experiences with regard to transrectal procedures, two of the men felt that these were neither that difficult to endure, and secondly, had little impact on their sense of masculinity:

> *We've got two friends who refused to be screened. They are terrified with what we have found and one of their fathers did have it. His father has just died – they're terrified about the finger up the bum bit too. OK it's not nice, but gee, if that's the worst thing that's ever going to happen to you in your life then you're not doing too badly. (6 years post-diagnosis, hormone treatment for secondary disease, 61–70 years)*

Another respondent comments:

> *The [digital rectal examination] might worry some guys but it didn't worry me at all. It's all over quickly and that's that. (6 months post initial treatment, organ-confined disease, 61–70 years)*

This was the approach that a distinct minority of the men took with regard to the transrectal procedures – that if it was needed, and it might help, then 'so be it'. It was considered an uncomfortable procedure that had no particular relevance to their identities or senses of masculinity. Despite the experiences of this small minority, investigative and diagnostic procedures were a source of considerable humiliation and degradation for these men – experiences that were closely tied to cultural codes of masculinity and the 'masculine ideal'. The location (within the range of the rectum) and function (delivery of semen) of the prostate makes an already difficult process (i.e. vulnerably, illness and thus weakness) even more problematic for these men's gendered identities.

TREATMENTS, SIDE EFFECTS AND MASCULINITIES

The implications of prostate cancer for masculinity are not confined to investigative or diagnostic procedures. Some of the most significant implications become prominent during and after treatment (Gray *et al.*, 2002; Kunkel *et al.*, 2000; Lucas *et al.*, 1995). The most common treatments for prostate cancer – the radical prostatectomy and radiation treatment – each carry considerable risks of impotency and incontinence (NCI, 2003; Stanford *et al.*, 2000). As suggested in the previous section, cultural ideals of masculinity are closely tied to heterosexuality (see Butler, 1990; Foucault, 1979), and particularly heterosexual penetration (potency) and desire, both of which may be difficult if not impossible after treatment.

The issue of potency represents an important, but often under-discussed factor for a significant number of men in decision-making processes (see also Gray *et al.*, 2000, 2002; Kunkel *et al.*, 2000). Emerging research in this area shows that, in the case of prostate cancer, potency is often not fully addressed in the decision-making process, becoming a major issue for men post-treatment (Gray *et al.*, 2000; Kunkel *et al.*, 2000). This is in part a result of the fact that medical specialists (and not just those in prostate cancer) have traditionally focused on cure or survival rates as central to treatment decisions. This is despite the fact that it is becoming increasingly apparent that some men are prepared to trade long-term survival for potency (Kunkel *et al.*, 2000). However, there is no data available on this issue and thus little is known about the influence of masculine ideas on men's treatment decisions. Thus, the current study explored these men's experiences of balancing 'cure' versus 'potency' and the role masculinity played in treatment decisions and experiences of treatment side effects.

Loss of potency, and its close links to dominant constructions of masculinity, arose as a significant issue for the majority of the men in this study:

> *Masculinity is an incredibly important thing. You know, my wife and I had reached a stage in our lives where sex had become really important. When we had the kids we were busy and sexual attraction waned but when I was 55 my boys were off at uni and we had some time to ourselves and we had matured sexually and it had become an important part of our lives. Now, we've never got that back [after the radical prostatectomy]. It [masculinity] varies from person to person. People's masculinity and their lovemaking is very different person to person. Masculinity is profoundly important. I've seen marriages break up from guys who have had a radical and never got back on deck with their potency and simply, it was the end of the marriage. The women said they couldn't cope – they needed to have that kind of lovemaking – only on one occasion did it break up a marriage but I've seen it create difficulties in quite a few marriages. (1–5 years post-treatment, organ-confined disease, 51–60 years)*

Loss of potency was talked about by several of these men as the most difficult aspect of their post-treatment stage. It was viewed as both impacting negatively on their well-being, and also, that of their wives. The possibility of losing potency also dominated the majority of these men's pre-treatment experiences. In particular, their desire to retain their sense of masculinity was omnipresent during the decision-making process and was an important factor in their final treatment decision. The prominence of masculinity as a factor was so influential for some of the men that the decision-making process was not about finding the best chance of 'cure', but rather, finding the treatment that would allow them to 'be a man' and retain the ability to perform sexually. As is captured in the excerpt below, several of the men specifically chose not to undergo a radical prostatectomy because they did not want to lose their sex life and sense of masculinity:

> *My sexual performance is very important, even to an older bloke like me, but so many people miss the point, that it's so much part of the male psyche; you*

take his manhood away from him and if it's been a thing that's important to him, and I have a whole long, long record of it being very important to me, if you take that away from the male, you change that male and that's not always understood – you change him entirely. So I opted for [treatment omitted to retain anonymity]. (1–5 years post-treatment, organ-confined disease, 61–70 years)

This respondent continues later in the interview:

Since I had the [treatment], when I met the first lady, that wanted to partake, and this was the first time after having the [treatment] and this is probably a couple of years after having the [treatment] and suddenly I was confronted with this lady who was quite keen to indulge, so having found a warm one ready to go one had to do something about it so I got hold of my GP and he briefed me on the injecting. It's a bit artificial but it works. The lady was ready to roll and I had to do something quick. The first time you do it it's a bit daunting because it's not something you really want to stick a needle into. However, if you handle it in all good humour you suddenly find that the result is worth the initial trial and actually it became quite a reasonable thing. (1–5 years post-treatment, organ-confined disease, 61–70 years)

This respondent provides a good example of the influence potency, and indeed, understandings of masculinity, may have on treatment decisions. Although retaining potency is clearly related to being able to partake in a pleasurable activity (regardless of its connection to 'being a man'), it is also closely linked to several of these men's gender identities. As suggested by one respondent: 'once the prostate has been removed … some men feel like they are no longer a complete man'. For several of the men interviewed here, the risk of not being 'a complete man' superseded the risk of death. In two cases, clearly 'inferior' treatments (in terms of its chance of cure) were chosen because of the potential to retain potency. The implication is that, in the case of prostate cancer, an already complicated process of selecting 'best' treatment (in terms of cure) is further complicated by the desire to retain the ability to 'be a man' or perform idealised forms of masculinity.

CONCLUSION

The aim of this chapter has been to embark on a critical exploration of the complex interplay between masculinities and prostate cancer, within the Australian context. It should be noted that the accounts presented here are those of a select group of men, and further research is needed to explore how experiences are mediated by other factors such as sexuality, geography, socio-economic status, ethnicity, and so on. However, given these limitations, within the accounts of these men there are important observations we can make about the intersectionality of masculinities and prostate cancer. Whilst there was significant heterogeneity in perspective amongst this group of men, the majority viewed biomedical investigations, disease and treatment processes as highly problematic in terms of their identities as men. Problems centred on the nature of the procedures (e.g. transrectal or exposure of the body) and the potential of treatments for taking away key components of the enactment of masculinity (e.g. potency and continence/control). These experiences seemed deeply embedded in a wider cultural idealisation of heterosexual masculinities, and were in turn enhanced by the perceived 'code of silence' surrounding illness and weakness within men's health cultures. It is not that having prostate cancer 'took away' or 'dissolved' their identity as a male, but rather reduced their ability to enact it and required a reformulation of self and identity (or indeed, selection of a treatment option less debilitating in terms of this enactment).

It was particularly interesting to note the tension between potential terminality and the desire to retain elements viewed as crucial to the enactment of masculine identity. Whilst it may be assumed by clinicians that desire to survive outdoes desire to 'perform', this may be at best oversimplistic. In fact, whilst more research is needed to confirm these findings, some of these men prioritised potency and lifestyle implications over cure, resulting in decision making that was deeply rooted in their desire to retain a sense of their identity as a male.

In light of the evidence presented here, it is crucial that all actors involved in the decision-making process (particularly the clinicians) are aware of the contradictory emotions faced by men within decision-making processes. Although negotiating dominant constructions of masculinity may not be difficult for some men in the face of a potentially life-threatening disease, the data presented here suggests that for others it will influence their choice of treatment and represents a major source of anxiety pre-, peri- and post-treatment. Allowing a non-pressurised, safe process in which men are able to communicate their values and priorities, rather than a process based on the simple assumption of 'cure' as isolated or uncomplicated, is essential for assisting men in the decision-making process. Furthermore, increasing the awareness of all parties regarding the impact that basic testing procedures may have on men's sense of masculinity is vital. The 'clinic' is a space in which gender is performed, and limiting the degree to which investigations disrupt men's performances of masculinity (i.e. avoiding 'shaming', ensuring privacy, maximising knowledge about procedure and the roles of particular health professionals) would likely limit the distress experienced by some men. Gaining an understanding of exactly how men experience such processes is essential for ensuring men are provided with adequate support and care pre-, peri- and post-treatment, and for facilitating community, carer and clinician awareness of the role masculinity plays in shaping men's experiences of disease.

NOTE

1 The 'happy needle' refers to local anaesthetic. In Australia, although it is officially subsidised by Medicare (the state health fund available to all Australians), urologists do not currently use anaesthetic during a prostate biopsy.

REFERENCES

AIHW (2007) *Cancer in Australia 2006*. Canberra: Australian Institute of Health and Welfare.

Broom, A. (2004) Prostate cancer and masculinity in Australian society: a case of stolen identity? *International Journal of Men's Health*, 3(2): 73–91.

Broom, A. (2005) The eMale: prostate cancer, masculinity and online support as a challenge to medical expertise. *Journal of Sociology*, 41(1): 87–104.

Broom, D. (2001) Reading breast cancer: reflections on a dangerous intersection. *Health*, 5(2): 249–68.

Butler, J. (1990) *Gender Trouble: Feminism and the Subversion of Identity*. London: Routledge.

Chapple, A. & Ziebland, S. (2002) Prostate cancer: embodied experience and perceptions of masculinity. *Sociology of Health & Illness*, 24(6): 820–41.

Connell, R.W. (2000) *The Men and the Boys*. St. Leonards, NSW: Allen & Unwin.

Connell, R.W (2005) *Masculinities* (2nd edn). Sydney: Allen & Unwin.

Courtenay, W. (2000) Constructions of masculinity and their influence on men's well-being: a theory of gender and health. *Social Science & Medicine*, 50: 1385–1401.

Foucault, M. (1977) *Discipline and Punish: The Birth of the Prison* (trans. A. Sheridan). London: Allen Lane.

Foucault, M. (1979) *The History of Sexuality*. London: Allen Lane.

Frydenberg, M. (1998) Management of localised prostate cancer: state of the art. *Medical Journal of Australia*, 169: 11–12.

Gray, R., Fitch, M., Fergus, K., Mykhalovskiy, E. & Church, K. (2002) Hegemonic masculinity and the experience of prostate cancer: A narrative approach. *Journal of Aging and Identity*, 7(1): 43–62.

Gray, R., Fitch, M., Phillips, C., Labrecque, M. & Fergus, K. (2000) To tell or not to tell: patterns of disclosure among men with prostate cancer. *Psycho-Oncology*, 9: 273–82.

Kiss, A. & Meryn, S. (2001) Effect of sex and gender on psychosocial aspects of prostate and breast cancer. *British Medical Journal*, 323(7320): 1055–9.

Korfage, I., Hak, T., de Koning, H. & Essink-Bot, M. (2006) Patients' perceptions of the side-effects of prostate cancer treatment: a qualitative interview study. *Social Science & Medicine*, 63: 911–19.

Kunkel, E., Bakker, J., Myers, R., Oyesanmi, O. & Gomella, L. (2000) Biopsychosocial aspects of orostate cancer. *Psychosomatics*, 41: 85–94.

Langellier, K.M. & Sullivan, C.F. (1998) Breast talk in breast cancer narratives. *Qualitative Health Research*, 8(1): 76–94.

Lucas, M., Strijdom, S., Berk, M. & Hart, G. (1995) Quality of life, sexual functioning and sex role identity after surgical orchidectomy in patients with prostatic cancer. *Scandinavian Journal of Urology and Nephrology*, 29(4): 497–500.

Lu-Yao, G., Albertsen, P., Stanford, J., Stukel, T., Walker-Corkery, E. & Barry, M. (2002) Natural experiment examining impact of aggressive screening and treatment on prostate cancer mortality in two fixed cohorts from Seattle area and Connecticut. *British Medical Journal*, 325(7367): 740.

Minichiello, V. (1995) *In-Depth Interviewing: Principles, Techniques, Analysis* (2nd edn). Melbourne: Longman.

NCI (2003) Prostate cancer. *National Cancer Institute*. http://www.cancer.gov/cancertopic/types/prostatecancer, accessed 25 March 2008.

Oliffe, J. (2004) Anglo-Australian masculinities and Trans Rectal Ultrasound Prostate Biopsy (TRUS-Bx): connections and collisions. *International Journal of Men's Health*, 3(1): 43–60.

Oliffe, J. (2005) Constructions of masculinity following prostatectomy-induced impotence. *Social Science & Medicine*, 60(10): 2240–59.

Oliffe, J. (2006) Embodied masculinity and androgen deprivation therapy. *Sociology of Health & Illness*, 28(4): 410–32.

PCFA (2008) Prostate cancer related statistics. *Prostate Cancer Foundation of Australia*. http://www.prostate.org.au, accessed 23 March 2008.

Potts, A. (2000) The essence of the hard on: hegemonic masculinity and the cultural construction of 'erectile dysfunction'. *Men & Masculinities*, 3(1): 85–105.

Rice, P. & Ezzy, D. (1999) *Qualitative Research Methods: A Health Focus*. Melbourne: Oxford University Press.

Robertson, S. (2006) 'I've been like a coiled spring this last week': embodied masculinity and health. *Sociology of Health & Illness*, 28(4): 433–56.

Stanford, J.L., Feng, Z., Hamilton, A.S. *et al.* (2000) Urinary and sexual function after radical prostatectomy for clinically localized prostate cancer: the Prostate Cancer Outcomes Study. *Journal of the American Medical Association*, 283: 354–60.

11 Understanding Masculinities within the Context of Men, Body Image and Eating Disorders

Murray Drummond

Introduction

It is arguable that men are somewhat underrepresented in the statistics associated with eating disorders and, in a broader sense, body-image concerns (Drummond, 1999, 2002a). Historically, eating disorders such as anorexia and bulimia nervosa have been identified as feminised conditions. That is, they have largely been associated with women and, in particular, adolescent females. The underpinning reason for such a notion has been the argument surrounding the pressure placed upon women to maintain a slim physique and one that is aesthetically appealing according to Western social and cultural archetypes (Rosenblum & Lewis, 1999; Tiggemann, 2001). It has been further identified that women have had to learn to adapt and live with such societal norms and, as a consequence, they adopt particular controlling behaviours associated with 'normative' bodily maintenance (Rosenblum & Lewis, 1999; Tiggemann, 2001). Up until recently such bodily maintenance was also regarded as a feminised ideal. However, as this chapter will identify, cultural evolution has placed enormous pressure on men, and in particular young men, to 'look' a certain way. That is, increasingly an archetypal body ideal based around athleticism, muscularity and being devoid of both body fat and hair, particularly the chest, back and shoulders, is perceived as being indicative of a dominant form of masculinity in contemporary Western culture (Drummond, 2005). Noteworthy, however, is that not all men perceive this new archetypal male physique as being the panacea to a masculine body identity. Indeed, there are certain groups of men who reject such a notion and who may even go out of their way to admonish this type of physique through personal behaviour such as overconsumption of food and alcohol and by verbally damning such physiques. The problem, however, is the backlash such men are now receiving through the dominant obesity discourse that pervades contemporary Western culture (Gard & Wright, 2005).

Contemporary Western society is not ideally set up to assist men with body-image concerns and eating disorders. Health professionals working in the area have few tools to help them in working with such men who may have a significant body-image concern, or an eating disorder at the very extreme, other than the resources and literature that focus on female eating disorders (Drummond, 2002a). While the manifestation of eating disorders is largely the same between genders there is a distinct and obvious difference in so far as we are dealing with men rather than women in this instance. Therefore issues associated with masculinities need to be taken into consideration and understood prior to working with men with eating disorders and body-image concerns. For example, understanding the importance of muscularity to the construction of one's masculine identity is critical, as too is situating the significance of sport and physical activity in men's lives. That is, *some* men's use of sport and physical activity as a means of weight loss must also be taken into consideration (Drummond, 1999, 2002a; Yates *et al.*, 1983). Further, some men who suffer from eating disorders and/or body image concerns may be attracted to certain sports and physical activities due to their highly controlled lifestyles (Drummond, 1996, 1999; Pope *et al.*, 2000; Yates *et al.*, 1983). For example, endurance sports such as marathon running or bodybuilding, both of which require immense physical demands.

This chapter will explore issues relating to masculinities and men's health with respect to body-image concerns among men. Essentially, the chapter is based upon interview data with various cohorts of men who express concern about their bodies and body image, including those men clinically diagnosed with eating disorders. It will also draw upon the literature in the field of men and masculinities, including the literature on men, sport and the body. I outline the research methodology to highlight the manner in which the study was grounded, then go on to identify and discuss major themes to illuminate some of the problematic issues surrounding men's bodies and eating disorders. Finally, I offer recommendations to assist practitioners working with body image-concerned and eating-disordered men.

MASCULINITY AND MEN IN THE CONTEXT OF HEALTH, BODY IMAGE AND EATING DISORDERS

Since the late 1990s there has been a significant increase in the number of research articles based around men's health and the social construction of masculinity (see for example Addis & Mahalik, 2003; Courtenay, 2000a, b; Riska, 2002; Robertson, 2006; Stibbe, 2004). Indeed, some of these articles, but certainly not all, pit men against women to highlight gender health inequities. The argument has often been based around the notion that the majority of men tend to access health services less than women and, as a consequence, men's health is generally poorer, particularly in terms of life expectancy (Courtenay, 2000a, b). There is also a strong cultural perception that men tend to deny or disguise symptoms associated with many illnesses until they become so serious as to jeopardise their quality of life (Courtenay, 2000a, b; Taylor et al., 1998).

This chapter is not designed to discuss the philosophical underpinnings of such an argument; suffice to say that for a range of reasons particular groups of men do not access health services as frequently as necessary to maintain health and longevity. However, with this in mind, coupled with the fact that some men struggle to come to terms with feminised illnesses and can feel embarrassed about seeking help for such conditions (Drummond, 1999, 2002a; Soban, 2006), the diagnosis and treatment of an illness such as a body image disorder or anorexia and bulimia nervosa is incredibly difficult among men (Soban, 2006).

SPORT AND PHYSICAL ACTIVITY IN THE CONTEXT OF MASCULINITIES, BODY IMAGE AND EATING DISORDERS

Sport and physical activity play a unique role in the social construction of masculinity among many men. Physical activity, particularly sport, is a highly masculinised domain (Drummond, 1996; Fitzclarence & Hickey, 2001; Messner, 1992). From an early age, boys are socialised to regard certain sports and physical activities as a rite of passage from boyhood into manhood. The sports that promote aggression and endurance are often seen as promoting masculine qualities (Young *et al.*1994). Social constructionist theorists have noted that those boys who do not become involved in 'masculine' sports can be marginalised from their peers (Whitson, 1990; Drummond, 1996, 2002b). Further, peers may taunt such boys as being less masculine or even label them as homosexual, gay, fags or sissy (Pronger, 1990; Messner, 1992; Epstein *et al.*, 2001).

A problematic issue within masculinised sporting and physical activity subcultures is the perpetuation and maintenance of masculine ideals that may be physically detrimental and injurious. Common for many men is the perception that enduring physical pain is part of what it means to be a man (Turner *et al.*, 2002). Therefore involvement in endurance sports is viewed as being a masculine pursuit. Events such as the Hawaii Ironman Triathlon in which competitors swim 3.8 km in open water, cycle 180 km and then run a full 42.2-km marathon, all in temperatures above 30°C have become symbolic of men's endurance sport, despite women being involved as well. Further, successful involvement in these activities is perceived as setting men apart from one another, thus creating a hierarchy of masculinities (Drummond, 1996; Messner, 1992). A large body of literature indicates that men can develop a sense of heightened masculinity through increased levels of muscularity (Mishkind *et al.*, 1986; Drewnowski *et al.*, 1995; O'Dea, 1995; Pope *et al.*, 2000; Choi *et al.*, 2002). As McCreary and Sasse (2000) see it, many men have a 'drive for muscularity' wherein they 'wish to be bulkier and more muscular than they currently see themselves' (p. 302). Paradoxically, the types of sports that promote endurance, and hence a form of masculine identity, generally require participants to be light in weight, with a consequent low level of 'muscular mesomorphy' (Mishkind *et al.*, 1986). The concept of 'doing' and 'being' (Drummond, 1996) therefore needs to be taken into consideration in this respect. That is, some men create a form of masculine identity through muscular body aesthetics, which could be argued as 'being'. Others perform masculinised 'acts' to enhance personal masculine identity. This may be contended as 'doing'. Take, for example, a successful Ironman triathlete's personal body image and perception of masculinity as opposed to that of a dedicated bodybuilder. The male triathlete is likely to gain his perception of masculinity through the success of competition and knowing that his body has competed to its fullest capacity. Despite not possessing a large body that occupies space to the same extent as that of a bodybuilder, there is contentment with regard to masculinity. Present is an awareness that his body is capable of performing, or *doing*, physical feats of endurance of which most men, including bodybuilders and women, are incapable. A body that is hard, lean and devoid of excess fat holds the endurance capacity to swim, cycle and run long distances for extended periods of time. Proud of his physiological health, this athlete displays accepted health-like qualities that are desired contemporary societal traits. To the Ironman triathlete, masculinity is perceived as a dynamic concept whereby masculine behaviours are developed through the performance and successful completion of regarded physical activities.

A bodybuilder, on the other hand, is different. Construction of masculinity is through the occupation of space and *being* hypermuscular, that is, the overdevelopment of a perceived masculine attribute. Together with this development is the manifestation of power which is displayed through physical prowess. Stronger and physically larger than any woman or average male, his physical presence is obtrusive. Dominance is established over anyone who is smaller and weaker and unable to match his size or strength, including peers in the weight room. Through bodybuilding this athlete has ultimately constructed a static form of masculinity. He has the *power of being*.

This *power of being* is not easily developed in bodybuilders and often comes at a price. Insecurity and powerlessness experienced by these men prior to their hypermasculine physiques is the price conferred upon them. In a discussion of a Californian bodybuilding subculture, Klein (1990), in his groundbreaking work, contended:

> The feelings of insecurity of many bodybuilders are often masked by veneers of power. The institution of bodybuilding not only makes a fetish of the look of power but also fosters identification with reliance upon figures of power. The claim here is that the institutionalised narcissism of bodybuilding, hypermasculinity, and homophobia is in part a reaction against feelings of powerlessness.
>
> (p. 241)

According to Klein (1990), it is the sense of powerlessness and the feeling of low self-worth that lead bodybuilders towards a craving for admiration. He claimed that 'in bodybuilding terms, admiration is dependent on building a powerful-looking physique and finding people to acknowledge it' (p. 130). However, it is contentious whether the physical power developed in bodybuilding equates to the type of kinaesthetic skill that is widely recognised as an intrinsic quality of *doing* sports. Messner (1992) highlighted this point by citing an interview with an ex-competitive runner who claimed that runners know

> *what speed their body's going at, they know how they are feeling, they have some sense of how much distance is left and what they can do, and very often will run against the clock, no matter what is going on in front of them; so they are not thrown off by people running foolishly fast or foolishly slow.*

> *(p. 63)*

Following an interview with a world-class, Australian surf life-saving Ironman, Connell (1990) argued that this top performer had a precise knowledge of his body and its capacities. It is this knowledge of their body, their kinaesthetic sense and the skill level at which they perform that sets these competitive *doing* sportsmen apart from the bodybuilder. Connell stated that the Ironman was quite eloquent about the particular kind of skill that was involved in top-level performance in his sport, and that it was far from being pure brawn. Such a statement is striking, since the suggestion of a typically masculine sport like the surf lifesaving Ironman being far from 'pure brawn' is a significant transformation or shift from the traditional masculine ideology and tenets of thought. In viewing 'endurance' sports as a physical activity to achieve a masculinised weight-loss goal (Drummond, 1998; Pope *et al.*, 2000; Yates, 1991), we can better understand why some men use physical activity to lose weight and body fat (Yates, 1991). Conversely, acts such as dieting are not perceived as appropriate weight-loss methods for men (Gough & Conner, 2006; Gough, 2007). The feminized stigma that is often linked to dieting may deter some men from food restriction or diet modification (Yates, 1991). When males simultaneously engage in sport and physical activity and restrict their food intake, they often do not generally acknowledge this combination as a primary weight-loss method (Drewnowski *et al.*, 1995; Yates, 1991). It appears that men tend to acknowledge exercise rather than food restriction and diet modification as a more 'masculine' model of weight control or loss (Drummond, 1999, 2002a; Yates, 1991). Schneider (1991) further reinforces this statement by claiming that 'it is more socially acceptable for a man to exercise than for a woman; "he's just a jock"' (p. 196).

There is a popular cultural perception within contemporary Western society that men are possibly somewhat immune to the problems that confront women in terms of eating disorders and associated body-image concerns. This has partially emerged as a response and 'cause' to fewer men being diagnosed with anorexia or bulimia nervosa (Drewnowski & Yee, 1987; Soban, 2006). It has also developed through the female-oriented perception of eating disorders, including the notion that cultural ideals place fewer constraints upon men with respect to body shapes and sizes (Drummond, 1999). Despite this common perception, there are men who suffer from anorexia and bulimia nervosa. Further, it is arguable that contemporary Western society produces an environment which places undue pressure on young men to 'look' a certain way in terms of youthfulness, muscularity and athleticism.

While one must be mindful that a variety of 'looks' do exist for young men and within specific contexts, this youthful, muscular, athletic body is tending to dominate Western cultural expectations of a masculinised body. This has emerged in close association with the gaze that now exists around men's bodies. Particularly in contemporary Western culture, the gaze associated with men's bodies may have never been stronger. Further, avenues of the gaze have intensified in terms of media focus, particularly with respect to advertising and popular culture television programmes. Increasingly men's bodies are being portrayed in ways that commercialise and objectify the male body in similar ways to how the female body has been, and remains, commodified. This, according to researchers, has played a significant role in the construction of negative body image in many men (Pope et al., 2000). I shall now attempt to highlight the concerns and experiences of some of these men by providing insight into their lives through rich life-historical accounts.

THE RESEARCH

The research that underpins this chapter has taken a similar approach with each of the groups of men. That is, the research is based on in-depth, qualitative interviews, utilising a life-historical perspective to capture the participant's reflections on their bodies from their earliest memories through to their current perceptions. A phenomenological approach has underpinned the research in so far as each of the research projects with the different groups of males has been based on the 'essence and meaning' (Patton, 2002) of what it is like to be a man with respect to the specific cohort in question. For example, what does it mean to be a man with an eating disorder? Similarly, what does it mean to be a gay man, or an adolescent boy growing up in contemporary Western society? The other groups of males to be researched have been ageing men, fitness leaders and elite-level athletes including surf lifesavers, triathletes and bodybuilders. Within the context of this research, the body has been the central focus with respect to the role it plays in the masculine identity of these males.

Clearly some of the participants, such as the eating-disordered men, had clinically diagnosed concerns with their bodies and body image, whereas other participants, despite seemingly comfortable with their body image and body identity, provided important information around the way in which the body comes to add to and detract from men's masculine identity. The stories of men from a range of ages and demographics therefore allow the reader to develop a sense of understanding of the issues confronting men, boys and their bodies. The themes highlighted within this chapter reflect the major issues confronting men with respect to body image.

Over 200 males have been involved in this research thus far. Each of the participants was selected on a voluntary basis. The interviews were carried out at convenient locations that enabled the participants to feel comfortable and at ease. As a consequence, most of the participants selected to be interviewed in cafés while others chose to be interviewed in their homes. All of the early adolescent schoolboys were interviewed at school, although some of the older adolescents chose to be interviewed somewhere away from the school environment, such as a café. Each interview lasted approximately one and a half to two hours, followed by shorter follow-up interviews, designed to gather any additional information required and as means of validity checks. An interview guide was utilised and was beneficial in allowing specific topics to be addressed. However, owing to the phenomenological nature of the research, the questions were essentially based on the participants' responses to previous questions. The interviews were transcribed verbatim and then coded and analysed accordingly using inductive thematic analysis. According to Patton (2002), inductive analysis allows for 'categories or dimensions to emerge from open-ended observations as the inquirer comes to understand patterns that exist in the phenomenon being investigated' (p. 56). Essentially, as Patton (2002) notes, this type of analysis involves identifying categories, patterns and themes in one's data through one's interaction with the data. Upon this analysis of the data, similarities and differences were documented based on my personal understanding, professional knowledge and the literature (Strauss, 1987). It should be noted that all of the research attained institutional Human Research Ethics Committee approval.

THEMES

In this section emergent themes will be presented to identify a variety of issues that influence the ways in which males perceive themselves and masculine identity with respect to their bodies. The emergent themes have been identified under the subheadings of the muscular male; fat consciousness; and men's bodies and the media: fitting the societal image.

The muscular male

Undoubtedly, the dominant theme to emerge from all of the interviews with males has been the notion associated with muscularity being a clear indicator of masculinity. The perception that muscularity equates to strength and that strength is a signifier of masculinity has also dominated the data. Therefore, the concept of looking formidable and dominant by 'being' muscular is an important aspect identified by most males across a range of ages. Similarly, 'doing' masculine acts using strength was inextricably linked to this notion. Therefore, when we consider issues associated with male body-image concerns it is important to be mindful of the archetypal representations of masculinity in contemporary Western culture. Indeed, this plays a significant role in the constructions of a male's masculine identity, given that visual endorsements of such cultural archetypes are constantly produced and reproduced in Western culture, archetypes to which many males aspire. An adolescent highlighted this by claiming:

> *The thing is, I am never happy with myself. I have always wanted to improve my body. I guess I find it's attractive to have a bigger body, you know, because people think, 'I don't want to start a fight with him because he's pretty big.*

While another adolescent affirmed:

> *I would like to be stronger, but then every guy would, so I can do more things. The more muscular you are, the more things you can do better. I guess that goes for all aspects of life.*

These types of comments are representative of what most of the males either claimed or alluded to. Even elite-level athletes, commonly perceived as cultural archetypal masculine heroes, held similar views and made comments on desiring more muscularity in order to positively impact their masculine identity. As one elite-level surf lifesaver stated:

> *I like myself. I like me, but I wouldn't mind being bigger. A bit bigger in size. Bigger in size, bit bigger in size. A bit heavier and a bit bigger in size. You know, blonde hair, blue eyes, tan. You know, your bronzed Aussie. That's a good look. I like that. I wouldn't mind being bigger. So, you know, I'm happy with myself but, if I could just be a bit bigger, I'd probably be a bit happier.*

Some of the males recognised the fact that they were never going to attain a culturally representative muscular, masculine physique. For example, the ageing men had reached a point in their lives where they were relatively happy with the way their bodies looked. However, they were far more concerned with the way their bodies were degenerating in terms of not be able to 'do' the physical tasks they were once capable of doing. Therefore, while not so concerned about appearance, they were concerned about diminishing performance and subsequent lack of masculine identity through reduced muscular strength. As one of the ageing men claimed:

> *When I was ill for 10 months, I used to be more physically fit and stronger, and I will never get it back like I used to. It makes me feel terrible, absolutely terrible. I could never understand my father-in-law, who used to be a boxer*

and was pretty fit, and he used to complain that he couldn't take a lid off a jar and he would get very upset that he physically could not do these things. And that was really upsetting. And that's the way I feel. I have physically lost things that my body just can't do.

While another man stated:

It affects me. The things I used to be able to do and I now can't do it. That really frustrates me. Some things I'm prepared to let go of, but others are much harder.

As these comments identify, body image is far more complex than merely a perception of one's body shape and whether it is a positive or negative association. These males clearly identify their body image as inextricably linked to what it can 'do', with muscularity and strength being key masculinised issues within this context. It is imperative that when thinking about men and their bodies we must be cognisant of the issues associated with the types of physical acts the body can and cannot do. At the same time we must also be mindful of the archetypal representations of the masculinised 'doing' body, and those who do and do not live up to those ideals.

Fat consciousness

The contemporary obesity discourse, which has medicalised and 'scientised' the terms 'overweight', 'fat' and 'obesity', has had a significant role in creating panic and uncertainty around body weight for the general community (Gard & Wright, 2005). The majority of males in these research projects, particularly the younger ones, raised issues pertaining to body fat. There is certainly a sense that fat is visually abhorrent on a contemporary archetypal male physique. Indeed, all of the eating-disordered males, as well as most of the adolescent ones, discussed this notion, together with the gay men and elite-level athletes. There was a strong perception by these men that developing and maintaining fatness was to display a lack of control, which in turn was not a masculine trait. As one young man claimed:

I would like to be a little bit skinnier. Not anorexic or anything. But you know, everywhere. Like some people can't find any fat anywhere, but I can when I pinch myself.

While another man stated:

I have cut back on food here and there. Sometimes after dinner I go to eat some more things and say to myself, 'I don't need this. I am going to live without it.

An eating-disordered male highlighted the abhorrence of fat by some contemporary males and, while at its extreme in this instance, reinforced the pressure to be devoid of its presence:

Like, it's fat. All the time. You know, you look in the mirror and you think, 'Oh, yuck'. It's either that or occasionally you might put on a little bit of weight and everyone will notice and that's when it really hits and you think, 'I've gotta lose weight, gotta lose weight'. That's what your mind is constantly telling you. Telling you to lose more weight. Break open some more stomach suppressants, whatever. Go on every diet there is. And do more exercise.

Certainly, this final quote is representative of an extreme form of body image disorder. However, I would argue that, over the 12 years I have been conducting interviews with males across a variety of ages and demographics, young males are becoming increasingly more concerned with body fat. Arguably, the most alarming aspect of this is that it is not based around notions of health. Rather, it is based on body aesthetics. The young men claim that body fat minimises the ability to see muscularity. Body-builders often talk about being 'ripped' and 'cut', which, interestingly, is the same vernacular used by many of the adolescent males throughout the research. Similarly, there is the additional issue of body hair, which is also seen by many younger males as thwarting the capacity of the muscular aesthetic. Indeed, some of the males have confirmed they shave or wax body parts to 'look more appealing'. However, the vexed question is, 'to whom?' The significant aspect of this is not in the exfoliation itself, rather the control it appears younger males have succumbed to according to bodily aesthetics. At a recent conference a female academic in the audience, and a mother of several girls, suggested that one would be forgiven for thinking that the above quotes emanated from girls and not young males. While I agreed, it highlights the notion that awareness of males and their aversion to body fatness is in its infancy, and is arguably not well understood. A primary issue of concern is based around where these males are constructing their ideologies with respect to bodily aesthetics.

Men's bodies and the media: fitting the societal image

Finally, the majority of males identified that, rightly or wrongly, the media play a significant role in the construction of the archetypal male physique. Further, they argued that media images have a far greater negative impact upon a male's sense of masculine identity than providing positive physiques to aspire to.

Several gay men articulated the perceptions of a majority of the research cohort when they quickly identified magazines as the major source of their frustration with respect to the exhibition of men's bodies. For example, one man stated:

> We are seeing a bit more fashion when it comes to television. Whereas the magazines and other media tend to be more naked, physical, your body. I was just thinking how media sets the standards for the rest of us as to what we see, what we accept and what we buy. Because you might think, 'he's pretty hot', but then you try to get that body and it just never happens.

Similarly, another participant claimed:

> Yeah. Like I used to buy them and I just stopped buying them because it made me depressed. You look at the guys in that magazine and they're all the perfect body and they're basically saying this is what you should look like if you want to go out and get a guy.

These types of comments were consistent across the majority of male participants. As a young heterosexual male claimed:

> Definitely the media play a big part. I think there are a lot of people in advertising who look good and other people see that and want to be like it.

Further, it was claimed that:

> We definitely get the images from the media. I think there are a lot of people in the magazines who look good and other people see that and want to be like it. I mean it's not just girls either. It's happening with guys too.

An overall summary was provided by one of the boys:

> Probably in this world, it does matter what your body looks like. Because it has an impact on you as a person, and you are judged by other people.

It is clear from the comments above that particular cohorts of young males are responding to the overt messages and images displayed in contemporary Western media. Some have referred to this media attention as a form of scrutiny and, as such, part of the contemporary male gaze (Bordo, 2000; Drummond, 2005). It is arguable that males have not had to endure such scrutiny in the past and are therefore struggling to come to terms with this phenomenon. Even for the younger males who may not have experienced the less gazed-upon era, and while seemingly accepting of such a new era, it is arguable that contemporary Western culture is not entirely sensitive to the needs of young men who do struggle with body-image concerns and eating disorders. It is further arguable that as result of this, as well as having less experience in working with males with such conditions, contemporary health practitioners may not be entirely equipped to assist males at the appropriate level. That being said, contemporary health practitioners are working within the parameters currently established for dealing with men, body-image and eating disorders. It is likely that a contextual and theoretical shift around the way in which body-image and eating disorders are developed among men will influence these parameters.

DISCUSSION

While the richness of the data provides tangible evidence of the way in which men reflect dominant ideologies of men's bodies and body image in contemporary Western culture, the relationship of these ideologies to masculinity is crucial in understanding their meaning and significance to men. Importantly, the themes identified in this chapter are those that are explicit, where the men have stated and discussed the issues within the context of in-depth individual interviews. It is the non-explicit themes such as the confusion surrounding what it is to be a man in contemporary Western culture that have not been identified. Most of the males interviewed struggled with defining the meaning of masculinity. It was notable that heterosexual males had more difficulty than young gay men in articulating the meaning of masculinity. For most of the heterosexual males, heterosexual masculinity was defined through size and shape of the body. Therefore, the 'being' notion played a significant role in their conceptualisation of contemporary masculinity. However, the simplest way in which heterosexual males defined masculinity was to identify *what it is not* (see also Gough, 1998). That is, not 'being' feminine in terms of having a small physique and not 'doing' feminine in terms of embracing culturally feminised behaviours and mannerisms.

Conversely, it was the gay men who had the capacity to articulate their meaning of masculinity in a far more fluid and reflective manner. Arguably these males have had to continually assess their masculine 'position' in society from a very early age and have therefore developed an ability to understand and interpret their sexuality, body and masculinity. It may be that young heterosexual males are provided with fewer opportunities to reflect upon their sexuality and masculinity given the culture in which they exist, which often reinforces a lack of introspection and personal care around heterosexual masculinity (Drummond, 2005).

Notwithstanding issues of sexuality and eating-disordered behaviour, it appears that of the male participants interviewed over the past 12 years the younger, adolescent, males are most critical of their bodies in terms of comparison with the archetypal male physique. Young men establishing their masculine identity through muscularity is a key component in this relationship. Interestingly, when discussing these issues with the ageing men the association between muscular aesthetics and masculinity is negligible. The importance of having a 'doing' functional body plays far more significance in these men's lives. Further, when the body can no longer 'do' the masculine acts and the men have come to terms with these changes, simply being alive is prioritised.

The archetypal male body has evolved and will continue to do so, based on the cultural standards that are prevalent at a particular time. According to the males that I have interviewed over the past 12 years, the current archetypal masculine male body has evolved into one which is muscular, yet not overly so. It is one that displays a degree of athleticism and hence has little visible signs of fatness. The terms 'ripped', 'cut' and 'chiselled' are terms that have been used frequently throughout the discussion on bodies with males. The terms represent masculinised discourse on a way in which the body should appear to others. They are also terms that reflect a 'doing' form of masculinity with respect to the associations with masculinised work. It is clear that the cultural evolution of the archetypal male body is closely aligned to media portrayals and representations of highly desirable male physiques. It is arguable that these physiques for males are as representative of the general male population as the cover girls in women's magazines are for females. Much has been written about this dilemma for women with respect to body image and the current similarities for males are striking, with the advent of the new men's magazine genre (Pope *et al.*, 2000). There is a need to address this situation now before men's body-image concerns become a *serious public health issue*. Therefore while there is evidence to indicate that men do develop eating disorders, it is arguable that a more insidious cultural phenomenon around masculine aesthetics is taking place. Just as the gaze upon women has created immense physical, mental and social concerns for this gender, there is a need to understand that men and their bodies are of contemporary cultural significance to minimise any harmful effects that may occur through the inevitable mounting gaze upon men. Additionally, such levels of understanding will better inform practitioners working with men who may have primary or secondary issues associated with body-image and eating disorders.

REFERENCES

Addis, M.E. & Mahalik, J.R. (2003) Men, masculinity, and the contexts of help seeking. *American Psychologist*, 58(1): 5–14.

Bordo, S. (2000) *The Male Body: A New Look at Men in Public and in Private*. New York: Farrar, Straus & Giroux.

Choi, P.Y., Pope, H.G., Jr & Olivardia, R. (2002) Muscle dysmorphia: a new syndrome in weightlifters. *British Journal of Sports Medicine*, 36: 375–6.

Commonwealth Department of Health and Human Services (1995) *Draft National Men's Health Policy*.

Connell, R.W. (1983) Men's bodies. *Australian Society*, 2(9): 33–9.

Connell, R.W. (1990) An iron man: the body and some contradictions of hegemonic masculinity. In M. Messner & D. Sabo (eds), *Sport, Men and the Gender Order: Critical Feminist Perspectives*. Champaign, IL: Human Kinetics, pp. 83–95.

Courtenay, W. (2000a) Constructions of masculinity and their influence on men's well-being: a theory of gender and health. *Social Science & Medicine* 50(10): 1385–401.

Courtenay, W. (2000b) Engendering health: a social constructionist examination of men's health beliefs and behaviours. *Psychology of Men and Masculinity*, 1(1): 4–15.

Drewnowski, A., Kurth, L. & Krahn, D. (1995) Effects of body image on dieting, exercise, and anabolic steroid use in adolescent males. *International Journal of Eating Disorders*, 17(4): 381–6.

Drewnowski, A. & Yee, D. (1987) Men and body image: are males satisfied with their body weight? *Psychosomatic Medicine*, 49: 626–34.

Drummond, M. (1996) 'The Social Construction of Masculinity as It Relates to Sport: An Investigation into the Lives of Elite Male Athletes Competing in Individually-Oriented Masculinised Sports'. Doctoral thesis, Edith Cowan University, Perth, Australia.

Drummond, M. (1998) When size matters: concerns and confusion over the ideal male body form. *National Body Image Conference proceedings*. Melbourne.

Drummond, M. (1999) Life as a male 'anorexic'. *Australian Journal of Primary Health Interchange*, 5(2): 80–9.

Drummond, M. (2002a) Men, body image and eating disorders. *International Journal of Men's Health*, 1(1): 79–93.

Drummond, M. (2002b) Sport and images of masculinity: the meaning of relationships in the lifecourse of male athletes. *Journal of Men's Studies*, 10(2): 129–41.

Drummond, M.J.N. (2005) Men's bodies: listening to the voices of young gay men. *Men and Masculinities*, 7(3): 270–90.

Epstein, D., Kehily, M., Mac an Ghaill, M. & Redman, P (2001) Boys and girls come out to play: making masculinities and femininities in school playgrounds. *Men and Masculinities*, 4: 158–72.

Fitzclarence, L. & Hickey, C. (2001) Real footballers don't eat quiche: old narratives in new times. *Men and Masculinities*, 4(2): 118–39.

Fletcher, R. (1992) *Australian Men and Boys: A Picture of Health?* Newcastle, NSW, Australia: University of Newcastle.

Gard, M. & Wright, J. (2005) *The Obesity Epidemic: Science, Morality and Ideology*. London: Routledge.

Gough, B. (1998) Men and the discursive reproduction of sexism: repertoires of difference and equality. *Feminism & Psychology*, 8(1): 25–49.

Gough, B. (2007) Real men don't diet: an analysis of contemporary newspaper representations of men, food and health. *Social Science & Medicine*, 64: 326–37.

Gough, B. & Conner, M.T. (2006) Barriers to healthy eating amongst men: a qualitative analysis. *Social Science & Medicine*, 62: 387–95.

Klein, A. (1990) Little big man: hustling, gender narcissism, and bodybuilding subculture. In M. Messner & D. Sabo (eds), *Sport, Men and the Gender Order: Critical Feminist Perspectives*. Champaign, IL: Human Kinetics, pp. 127–39.

McCreary, D.R. & Sasse, D.K. (2000) An exploration of the drive for muscularity in adolescent boys and girls. *Journal of American College Health*, 48: 297–304.

Messner, M. (1992) *Power at Play*. Boston, MA: Beacon Press.

Mishkind, M.E., Rodin, J., Silberstein, L.R. & Striegel-Moore, R.H. (1986) The embodiment of masculinity: cultural, psychological, and behavioural dimensions. *American Behavioural Scientist*, 29: 545–62.

O'Dea, J. (1995) Body image and nutritional status among adolescents and adults: a review of the literature. *Australian Journal of Nutrition and Dietetics*, 52: 56–67.

Olivardia, R., Pope, H.G., Jr & Hudson, J.I. (2000) Muscle dysmorphia in male weightlifters: a case-control study. *American Journal of Psychiatry*, 157: 1291–6.

Patton, M. (2002) *Qualitative Research and Evaluation Methods* (3rd edn) Thousand Oaks, CA: Sage.

Pope, H., Phillips, K. & Olivardia, R. (2000) *The Adonis Complex: The Secret Crisis of Male Body Obsession*. New York: Free Press.

Pronger, B. (1990) *The Arena of Masculinity: Sports, Homosexuality, and the Meaning of Sex.* New York: St. Martin's Press.

Riska, E. (2002) From Type A man to the hardy man: masculinity and health. *Sociology of Health & Illness,* 24(3): 347–58.

Robertson, S. (2006) 'I've been like a coiled spring this last week': embodied masculinity and health. *Sociology of Health & Illness,* 28(4): 433–56.

Rosenblum, G.D. & Lewis, M. (1999) The relations among body image, physical attractiveness and body mass in adolescence. *Child Development,* 70(1): 50–64.

Schneider, J. (1991) Gender identity issues in male bulimia nervosa. In C. Johnson (ed.), *Psychodynamic Treatment of Anorexia Nervosa and Bulimia.* New York: Guilford Press, pp. 194–222.

Soban, C. (2006) What about the boys? Addressing issues of masculinity within male anorexia nervosa in a feminist therapeutic environment. *International Journal of Men's Health,* 5(3): 251–67.

Stibbe, A. (2004) Health and the social construction of masculinity in *Men's Health* magazine. *Men and Masculinities,* 7: 31–51.

Strauss, A. (1987) *Qualitative Analysis for Social Scientists.* Cambridge: Cambridge University Press.

Taylor, C., Stewart, A. & Parker, R. (1998) 'Machismo' as a barrier to health promotion in Australian males. In T. Laws (ed.), *Promoting Men's Health: An Essential Book for Nurses.* Melbourne: Ausmed Publications, pp. 14–29.

Tiggemann, M. (2001) Children's body image: it starts sooner than you think. *Virtually Healthy,* 19:3, pp. 1–2.

Tolson, A (1987) *The Limits of Masculinity.* London: Routledge.

Turner, A., Barlow, J. & Ilbery, B. (2002) 'Play hurt, live hurt': living with and managing osteoarthritis from the perspective of ex-professional footballers. *Journal of Health Psychology,* 7(3): 285–301.

Whitson, D. (1990) Sport in the social construction of masculinity. In M. Messner & D. Sabo (eds), *Sport, Men and The Gender Order: Critical Feminist Perspectives.* Champaign, IL: Human Kinetics, pp. 19–29.

Yates, A. (1991) *Compulsive Exercise And Eating Disorders: Toward an Integrated Theory Of Activity.* New York: Brunner/Mazel.

Yates, A., Leehy, K. & Shisslak, C. (1983) Running – an analogue of anorexia nervosa? *New England Journal of Medicine,* 308(5): 251–5.

Young, K., White, P. & McTeer, W. (1994) Body talk: male athletes reflect on sport, injury, and pain. *Sociology of Sport Journal,* 11: 175–94.

12 THE ROLE OF MASCULINITIES IN WHITE AND SOUTH ASIAN MEN'S HELP-SEEKING BEHAVIOUR FOR CARDIAC CHEST PAIN

Paul Galdas

INTRODUCTION

Empirical data are increasingly bearing out theorised connections between the construction of hegemonic masculinities and men's poor help-seeking practices. Several studies have implicated hegemonic masculinities as having a detrimental effect on how men manage the impact of conditions such as prostate cancer on their life, particularly in relation to expressing emotion and seeking emotional support (Lavery & Clark, 1999; Gray *et al.*, 2000; Broom, 2004; George & Fleming, 2004; Oliffe, 2005). In one such study, Chapple and Ziebland (2002) found that, among 52 men diagnosed with prostate cancer in the UK, many had been hesitant about seeking help for their problems because they believed it was not 'macho' to seek advice about health problems, that 'boys don't cry', and it was not 'masculine' to display signs of weakness. Recent research involving men with depression (Emslie *et al.*, 2006), as well as healthy men (O'Brien *et al.*, 2005; Robertson 2006), has also indicated that those who adhere to hegemonic versions of masculinity are reluctant to discuss health problems with others; only contemplate seeking help following pain, endurance, stoicism and visible injury; and need a means of legitimising their visit to a doctor to keep their male identity intact.

Delays in seeking medical treatment have a significant impact on disease progression. This is especially true in coronary heart disease (CHD). CHD is the leading cause of premature death for men worldwide, and clinical trials have shown that the most critical factor in preventing premature death from CHD is rapid access to medical treatment within 12 hours of symptom onset (GISSI, 1986, 1995; ISIS-2, 1988; UKHAS, 1998). Survival from cardiac arrest may be trebled by improving men's and women's help-seeking response to their CHD symptoms (Norris, 1998). However, few researchers have provided an explicitly gendered analysis of men's experiences of seeking help for the symptoms of an acute cardiac condition (Emslie, 2005). A qualitative investigation conducted by White and Johnson (2000) is the only study to date that has explored men's interpretations of cardiac-related chest pain and considered the impact of masculinity on their help-seeking process. White and Johnson (2000) studied 20 men admitted to a coronary care unit in the UK and found that most had been reluctant to seek medical help, despite having suffered severe, debilitating chest pain. Akin to the themes identified in the studies discussed earlier, several men in White's investigation explained that they had been reluctant to discuss their health problems with others because they feared appearing a 'wimp' or 'unmanly'. White and Johnson (2000) explained men's reticence to seek medical help as a result of their continuous assessment of their performance against society's expectations of them as men; a performance which is threatened by the possibility of ill health and leads to the use of denial as a psychological defence:

> It seems that man [sic] is not prepared to deal with his body when it makes the transition from being healthy to being ill. He is expected to be fit, productive and able to carry out the roles expected of him. There is a feeling of invincibility that is deep-seated and, when this is threatened, men have to rationalise their position and negotiate ... about what to do. (p. 540)

Delays in accessing prompt and appropriate medical help for the symptoms of CHD have particularly serious implications for the health of men of South Asian ethnicity. Patterns of CHD morbidity and mortality vary among men of differing ethnicity. Numerous studies of migrant South Asian populations living in Western countries – defined as those born in India, Pakistan or Bangladesh – have confirmed higher rates of CHD compared with other ethnic and migrant groups (Sheth et al., 1999; Yusuf et al., 2001, 2004; Joshi et al., 2007). In the UK, for example, the premature death rate from CHD is 46 per cent higher in South

Asian men compared with the white indigenous population (British Heart Foundation, 2005). Yet, despite the immense CHD burden among the migrant South Asian male population and growing evidence pointing toward the deleterious effect of masculinity on men's health and help-seeking behaviour, the issue of masculinities and their impact on both white and South Asian men's help-seeking behaviour for the symptoms of CHD has received little research attention.

As discussed earlier in this book, the pluralising of masculinity – the recognition of multiple masculinities – has been a central tenet of the social-constructionist gender framework. Connell's (2005) influential work contrasted culturally authoritative, hegemonic patterns of masculinity with less powerful configurations of gender practice. The framework emphasises that other masculinities coexist, or more precisely are produced at the same time as hegemonic masculinities. These include marginalised masculinities: gender forms produced in exploited or oppressed groups, such as ethnic minorities (Connell, 2005). Yet, despite this complexity, with some notable exceptions (Emslie *et al.*, 2006; Robertson, 2006), masculinity has often been essentialised and reduced to a singular construct by men's health researchers – the stereotypical white, middle-class, heterosexual man – and deployed in relation to the association between masculinity and health (Gough, 2006). The aforementioned studies on men's help-seeking behaviour, both empirically and theoretically, predominantly embody a distinctly white, Western male perspective of masculinity (Galdas *et al.*, 2005; Oliffe *et al.*, 2007).

Addressing this gap in the body of knowledge, this chapter presents data from in-depth interviews with 36 white men and 20 South Asian (Pakistani and Indian) men admitted to two UK hospitals with the symptoms of an acute cardiac event. Men's experiences of interpreting, and acting upon, their CHD symptoms are explored, and the extent to which configurations of gender practice intersected with their help-seeking behaviours and decision-making are examined.

METHODS

Grounded theory methods (described in detail elsewhere – see Galdas *et al.* [2007]) were used to investigate the process involved in the decision to seek or delay seeking medical help and the interrelationship of this process with men's constructions of masculinity. The study participants were all hospital inpatients who had experienced chest pain and had a confirmed (new) diagnosis of CHD. Fifty-six men took part in the study: 36 white men and 20 South Asian men of Indian or Pakistani origin. Participants' ethnicity was self-determined according to ancestry (family origins). Only three participants in the study were not married: two white men (participants 8 and 48) were cohabiting with long-term female partners and one white man (participant 5) was single and lived alone. The Indian and Pakistani participants were a heterogeneous group in terms of religious affiliation (Muslim, Sikh and Hindu), and all but one (participant 47) had been born and educated in the Indian subcontinent and had migrated to the UK during the previous 30 years. Delay in help-seeking, defined as time taken from first onset of chest pain to the call for medical help (as documented in medical records and verified by participants during interview), varied between less than one hour to more than seven days.

RESULTS

Men's accounts of their experiences illustrated that the decision to seek medical help was a complex process mediated by a number of factors including age, context of the event (e.g. at home, in the workplace), past medical history, occupation and knowledge of symptoms. In this chapter, three key themes that emerged from the data in relation to the role of masculinity in white and South Asian men's decisions to seek or delay seeking medical help are discussed. These are: the symbolic status of chest pain, disclosing pain to others, and use of primary healthcare services.

The symbolic status of chest pain

At the onset of symptoms, men had attempted to make sense of what was causing their chest pain to determine what action, if any, needed to be taken. Pain was initially attributed to a non-serious condition, such as indigestion or trapped wind. Whether medical help was considered necessary was determined after a period of waiting to see if the pain became worse. Although men's responses towards their chest pain during the early stages of onset were similar, there were marked differences between how white and South Asian men reacted to their pain as it persisted.

The need to display a high threshold for pain and discomfort was important to white men in the study. This was illustrated by several men expressing a fear of being seen to be weak by friends, relatives or health-care professionals if they sought medical help for pain that was perceived to be 'tolerable'. As one man noted:

> To the ambulance men I said, 'Look, I kept on going to work'. My wife kept saying, 'You're not a softy' and probably I had some in-built thing like, you know, they will be saying, 'Oh it's just a little pin-prick', that sort of thing ... I was trying to convey to them that I'm not a softy, I don't get upset at the slightest thing. (Participant 46; 49-year-old white male; delayed seeking help for three hours)

Men who had experienced chest pain at work were concerned that colleagues would view them as hypochondriacs or as 'swinging the lead' if they sought help. From the accounts of the majority of white men it was clear that these perceptions had played a part in their decisions to delay seeking medical help.

Not all white men's experiences were consistent with this pattern of behaviour. Three men (identified as 'negative cases') told of how they had *immediately* left work and sought medical help at the onset of their symptoms. For example, one man, a 57-year-old security guard (participant 7), had been trained in first aid and was aware of the symptoms of MI. He experienced the onset of his chest pain at work, immediately associated his symptoms with a heart problem and went straight to the casualty department of a local hospital. Comparable accounts were given by a hospital worker and a man whose father had recently died of a heart attack. All three men explained that their knowledge of heart disease had led them to be confident about the seriousness of their chest-pain symptoms. However, the men were also keen to assert their high tolerance for pain during their interview. Participant 7, for instance, stressed that the reason he had sought help promptly for his chest pain was not because he could not tolerate the pain, but rather, because he *knew* his condition was serious. Indeed, it was clear from most white men's narratives that the majority had *not* considered their chest pain to be worthy of medical attention until it became incapacitating or until they experienced additional symptoms, such as breathlessness, sweating or pallor:

I can usually diagnose myself. If I think I can do. I'd rather do that than go to the doctor ... and just leave it. But this [chest pain], I knew there was something there, so that was why I came straight up [to the hospital]. (Participant 7; 57-year-old white male; delayed seeking help for less than 1 hour)

After breakfast, getting into the car it felt a bit tight in my chest, but nothing disastrous. It wasn't something that was going to cause me any trouble. I've got a high pain tolerance ... but I got to work, did a couple of e-mails, sorted a couple of things out and I thought, the rest of the work I've got today I can do at home, and I thought I don't feel that great, I'll go work at home and it was still there, and I then just felt clammy and I thought well, it must be something. (Participant 16; 57-year-old white male; delayed seeking help for 12 hours)

By comparison, the experience of prolonged chest pain caused greater anxiety in Indian and Pakistani men, and the main cause of help-seeking delay appeared to be a failure to promptly attribute symptoms to the heart. However, most Indian and Pakistani participants had considered their pain to be a legitimate reason to seek medical help when they realised it was persistent and/or recurrent. Moreover, no Indian or Pakistani man considered seeking help for their chest pain to be 'unmanly' or a sign of weakness. When questioned about what they did consider to be valued male attributes, several men placed great emphasis on wisdom, education and responsibility for the family and one's health.

If you are an educated person, naturally you will seek some advice from the doctor. In the Asian men I have seen if they are [ill] they all go to see their doctors ... It's different here [in England]. (Participant 56; 52-year-old Pakistani Muslim male; delayed seeking help for 6 hours)

Very strong the man that works for others, lives for others, lives for their own self ... but they must also live for others. Family, first family and then others, so you must visit the doctor. (Participant 55; 72-year-old Pakistani Muslim male; delayed seeking help for 4 hours)

If that pain I had never had it before and it was very new and I don't know and it was causing serious, I would go to doctor definitely rather than pretending there is no problem. For example, flu is common problem for me and if it happens I normally don't go to doctor because from childhood this is problem for me, so I know already. I know that whenever it starts it goes and after two or three days, but if it is something new I would definitely go to the doctor ... Every wise man knows what he should do, for example, I am an educated person. I know these are very basic logical things. I should know what I should do in that situation [when experiencing chest pain]. That is a logical decision. (Participant 1; 48-year-old Pakistani Muslim male; delayed seeking help for 4 hours)

Disclosing pain to others

The differing meanings men attributed to their chest pain strongly influenced their decisions whether to disclose their symptoms to others. The majority of Indian and Pakistani men had discussed their symptoms with family members. These discussions often led to an endorsement that their pain was significant and worthy of medical attention:

I talked to my brother about it, he told me this reaction [to seek medical help] ... so I see the doctor but not panic. (Participant 55; 72-year-old Pakistani Muslim male; delayed seeking help for 4 hours)

The family knew first. They push me ... my wife will and the children. There's nothing embarrassing [about seeking help]. If the doctor is needed you must go, they will push it. It doesn't seem more in the English families ... they don't discuss much with the family first. (Participant 38; 54-year-old Pakistani Muslim male; delayed seeking help for 6 hours)

In stark contrast, it was common for the majority of white men to describe disclosing their chest pain to others as being a last resort. Most had only disclosed their symptoms, usually to their wives/partners, when they could no longer tolerate the pain and felt confident it was a 'legitimate' illness that was worthy of concern. For example, one white man (participant 48) who experienced transient chest pain for almost two days while on holiday had kept it hidden from his partner until it eventually prevented him from walking. Others echoed similar feelings. Participant 50, for example, described how he had kept his symptoms hidden from his wife despite having recurrent chest pain for over 3 days:

I'm trying to think that hopefully it will just go away and in the end, when I told her, she [partner] insisted that I come down and I agreed because I was getting concerned myself ... In the first instance I usually keep things to myself, but eventually you seek another source, which in this case was my girlfriend. (Participant 48; 47-year-old white male; delayed seeking help for 36 hours)

I didn't tell her what happened Monday, Tuesday, Wednesday, I never told her about all these pains I'm having ... I just got on with it. (Participant 50; 55-year-old white male; delayed seeking help for 96 hours)

These differences between white and South Asian men's help-seeking behaviour were discussed in detail by two Pakistani men who talked about the contrast between stoic 'English' male behaviour and an 'Asian' male tendency to discuss and disclose illness to the family:

Not to tell anybody, that's not Asian, that's English ... [white English] men have this private, 'Oh I can deal with this myself'. (Participant 47; 46-year-old Pakistani Muslim male; delayed seeking help for 6 hours)

Use of primary health care services

All Indian and Pakistani participants, apart from one, had visited their general practitioner (GP) before being admitted to hospital. It was clear from these men's narratives that their reasons for consulting their GP were not only a means of seeking treatment, but were also an accustomed way of making sense of the meaning of symptoms.

I feel pain for long time. I thought I should have to go to my GP and he tell me what the pain is when I tell him so and so, pain in my chest and my arm ... when I came to the hospital, the doctor told me that they'd check me for a, you know this, the heart, there might be a problem, and I was a bit surprised to hear that. (Participant 39; 48-year-old Pakistani Muslim male; delayed seeking help for 4 hours)

I understand that you don't need an invitation to go to a doctor. If you are ill yourself, if you are ill and you want to keep it to yourself no one is going to help you. (Participant 49; 53-year-old Indian Hindu male; delayed seeking help for 1 hour)

Although religious beliefs did not emerge as a strong theme in the data, one Muslim man who was a retired GP of Pakistani origin suggested that Islam may be an important factor underpinning Muslim men's willingness to seek help from their doctor. He noted:

Even the Muslims in their religion they say 'If you are sick, seek a doctor, go to the doctor'. ... In the Holy book, the Prophet himself, he goes to the doctor, he got the medicine, he treated himself and he had to seek medicine, so every Muslim man knows about it. (Participant 53; 84-year-old Pakistani Muslim male; delayed seeking help for 1 hour)

By contrast, white men held a distinctly different perspective on access to primary health care and many talked with pride about the length of time since their last visit to their GP. Only one of the white participants had consulted a GP prior to their admission to hospital. Avoiding being perceived to be a hypochondriac or weak by others played a part in many white men's decision to delay seeking help from a health-care professional until they became certain their pain could not be coped with alone. When they had eventually sought medical help their condition usually necessitated admission to an accident and emergency department, not a GP visit. In contrast to the Indian and Pakistani men who appeared to be willing to consult their GP to make sense of their chest pain, seeking medical help was perceived by most white men to be a last resort. In an extreme case one white man who had delayed seeking help for almost three days drove to hospital rather than visit his GP or phone an ambulance. He was later diagnosed with an anterior myocardial infarction. When asked why he had chosen to drive himself to hospital rather than call an ambulance, he explained:

I don't want an ambulance coming up the bloody street and all that. I don't want people to think I'm poorly, you know what I mean … I just don't want pity, people looking'. (Participant 50; 55-year-old white male; delayed seeking help for 96 hours)

So I thought I'd set off to work. I mean I didn't feel too bad, I wasn't in agony, if I'd have been in agony I wouldn't have gone but there was some pain there … I mean I do go to the doctor's but it's not something I readily look to do, so I think sometimes if you can put things off you do tend to do that. (Participant 54; 57-year-old white male; delayed seeking help for 36 hours)

Interestingly, one South Asian participant did talk of reluctance to take time off work and seek medical help. The 46-year-old Pakistani Muslim man was the only participant in the study who had been educated in the UK as a child. He delayed seeking help for over 6 hours despite experiencing severe, intermittent central chest pain. His narrative clearly illustrated that he had only considered his symptoms to be worthy of medical attention once his breathing became erratic. He stressed the importance of maintaining his identity as a 'leader' at work and a desire to not appear weak to his work colleagues; perceptions he recognised as contributing to his decision to postpone seeking help during his experience of chest pain. Furthermore, he explained he had also been reluctant to allow his family to visit him when he was first admitted to hospital because he did not want them to see he was ill. Later in his interview, he revealed that recollecting the experiences of three football managers who had suffered heart problems recently had affirmed his decision that it was legitimate for him to call an ambulance.

I'd thought that, 'I'm a businessman, I can deal with this myself'. … But I'd read about people, sort of [football] managers going into hospital like Houllier and Souness and some of the others and in fact just recently when my home team thrashed the opposition 6–1, one of the managers … went into hospital for something else [to do with the heart] and I thought, that was the reason that prompted me to sort of call the ambulance. You know, best get it checked. (Participant 47; 46-year-old Pakistani Muslim male; delayed seeking help for 6 hours)

DISCUSSION

Beliefs about health and illness, and the meanings attributed to symptoms, have long been recognised as owing much to people's cultural beliefs and attitudes (Radley, 1994). In particular, there is a considerable body of evidence that asserts pain perception, and the behaviours associated with pain are primarily influenced by sociocultural factors (Bates, 1978; Berry, 1998; Montes-Sadoval, 2000; Nayak et al., 2000; Callister, 2003). For example, in a classic study of Italian, Jewish and 'Old American' men's reactions to pain, Zborowski (1952) found distinct differences between the different ethno-cultural groups. Italians appeared to complain about the pain itself, Jewish patients typically expressed worries about the implications of the pain on their health, and 'Old Americans' did not complain about their pain or display their feelings. Zborowski (1952) interpreted these various behavioural responses to pain in terms of men's different cultural attitudes as to what is acceptable as a way of complaining and seeking help. Similarly, the meanings men attribute to the symptoms of ill health, and their cultural attitudes as to what is gender-appropriate help-seeking behaviour, can be seen to signify social constructions of masculinity. To illustrate, in Western cultures, ideals of hegemonic masculinity embody the perception of men as 'naturally' strong, resistant to disease, unresponsive to pain and physical distress, and unconcerned with minor symptoms (Courtenay, 2000). Consistent with these ideals, most white men in this study had faced risk and physical discomfort rather than promptly engage in help-seeking behaviour which was viewed as emasculating, feminised, and symbolically assimilated with being a hypochondriac or weak. The men's narratives emphasised that seeking help or admitting the need for help – either from their wife, colleague or health-care professional – was a last resort. Indeed, it was not until the onset of additional physical symptoms, such as clamminess, breathlessness or loss of skin colour, or the onset of severe debilitating pain, that these men began to change their perception of their symptoms, consider their illness as 'legitimate', and accept that they required assistance. Thus, the accounts of white participants in this study cohere with a growing body of evidence which, as noted in the introduction to this chapter, exemplifies the intersections between the construction of hegemonic masculinities and men's poor help-seeking practices (Galdas *et al.*, 2005).

However, in contrast to previous studies, and those investigations that have suggested that men from ethnic minorities (living in Western societies) may also use signifiers of hegemonic masculinity – 'protest' or 'hyper' masculinities – in an attempt to protect and defend a compromised masculine identity (Franklin, 1984; Majors & Billson, 1992; Hearn & Collinson, 1994; Mac an Ghaill, 1994; Rich & Stone, 1996; Evans *et al.*, 2005), the majority of Indian and Pakistani men in this study appeared to have had acted in a way that was consistent with dominant South Asian representations of masculinity in the context of seeking medical help for chest pain. Most men emphasised that a willingness to seek prompt medical help (usually from the GP) when experiencing chest pain was an appropriate behaviour *for an Indian or Pakistani man*. Previous investigations of intersections of ethnicity and masculinities have predominantly investigated men who were born and socialised within a Western country; for example, Evans *et al.*'s (2005) study of men of Afro-Canadian men with prostate cancer. For these men, Western hegemonic (white male) constructions of masculinity can be considered to have been the dominant, culturally exalted representation of 'real manhood' throughout their lives. As Evans *et al.* (2005) note, historically, avenues for demonstrating masculinity have therefore been narrowed for black and ethnic minority men in Western culture. Our study sample was unusual because all but one participant had migrated to the UK as an adult. This may explain why, contrary to these previous findings, our results indicated that despite living in the UK the men did not perceive a need to use signifiers of Western hegemonic masculinity to defend their masculine identity. Several studies on medical help-seeking behaviour in India and Pakistan have found men are more willing and likely to seek medical help than women for a number of conditions (Nair *et al.*, 2002; Grover *et al.*, 2003; Morankar & Weiss, 2003; Atre *et al.*, 2004; Shaikh & Hatcher, 2005). This would suggest that the Indian and Pakistani men in this study aligned themselves with dominant South Asian ideals of masculinity when experiencing chest pain wherein – contrary to Western hegemonic masculine practices – seeking medical help is a dominant, male gender-appropriate behaviour.

Current prevailing gender-theoretical frameworks would position the South Asian men's constructions of masculinity in this context as being 'marginalised'; that is, their behaviour as a man (seeking help promptly) is perceived as 'weak' and devalued in Western cultures because it is not consistent with the pattern of behaviour culturally exalted as representing 'real' manhood (acting stoical, enduring pain, delaying seeking medical help, and so forth) (Courtenay, 2000; Connell, 2005). However, this study raises questions about whether, contrary to these prevailing gender frameworks, more than one representation of hegemonic masculinity can coexist in a given context and, specifically, that Western hegemonic representations of masculinity may in fact be only one of many culturally specific 'hegemonic reference points' around which masculinity is organised and adopted in the context of seeking medical help (Wall & Kristjanson, 2005). It was clear that most Indian and Pakistani men in our study did not perceive a need or expectation to conform to the Western hegemonic ideal. Furthermore, the men refuted strongly that others (such as wives, friends and colleagues) would view them as weak or less 'manly' as a result. These themes indicate that, despite living in a Western culture, most South Asian men in our study did not consider Western hegemonic representations of masculinity to be – as current social-constructionist gender frameworks assert

(Kimmel 1996; Courtenay, 2000; Connell, 2005) – the masculinity that 'sets the standards' for all other men in the context of
medical help-seeking. Defining South Asian men's masculinity as
being 'marginalised' (a concept primarily informed by studies of
the experiences of black/African-Caribbean men) may therefore
reflect an overly simplistic and ethnocentric masculine typology.
As Hearn and Collinson (1994) have argued, multiple masculinities are likely to be constructed through the various positioning of
the self and others with regard to interconnected social divisions
of gender, ethnicity and class, and some aspects of identity – such
as being Indian, Pakistani, a husband, a father, a business leader –
are likely to be prioritised over others in differing contexts. The
findings indicated that most participants prioritised their identity
as a South Asian man, and thus South Asian representations of
hegemonic masculinity, in the context of seeking medical help for
chest pain in the UK.

Interestingly, the experience of the only South Asian participant
in our study who had been educated in the UK prompts questions
about potential differences in the influence of masculinities on
the decision to seek medical help between South Asian men who
have migrated to the UK as an adult and the so called 'second
generation' who have been raised and socialised in the UK. Consistent with previous studies on white men's help-seeking behaviours that have identified being 'strong and silent', enduring pain,
and delaying seeking medical help as key practices of masculinity
(Gascoigne & Whitear, 1999; White & Johnson, 2000; Chapple &
Ziebland, 2002; Broom, 2004; Galdas et al., 2005; O'Brien et al.,
2005; Robertson, 2006), he noted that he had an 'English' men-
tality that corresponded to a perceived need to hide his pain from
his friends and family due to a fear of being seen to be 'weak'.
Moreover, his perception of himself as a 'businessman' and 'leader'
points towards factors such as socio-economic status that may play
a crucial role in South Asian men's construction of masculine
identity in the context of help-seeking. This aspect of his account
is consistent with a central tenet of constructing hegemonic masculinities in Western industrialised capitalist societies that embody
the perception of men primarily as 'breadwinners' (Connell,
2005), pointing towards relationships between 'localised' hegemonic forms of masculinity and 'international' forms such as those
outlined in Connell's work on globalised masculinities (Connell,
2000; Connell & Messerschmidt, 2005). Connell argues that while

local forms of hegemonic masculinity may differ, they are, or will be, increasingly subject to the global hegemonic norm. The study discussed in this chapter highlights the need for further research with men of South Asian descent, who have been born/raised and educated in Western countries, to further develop this theory and examine in detail how ethnicity interplays with men's configurations of gender practice in the context of seeking medical help.

REFERENCES

Atre, S.R., Kudale, A.M., Morankar, S.N., Rangan, S.G. & Weiss, M.G. (2004) Cultural concepts of tuberculosis and gender among the general population without tuberculosis in rural Maharashtra, India. *Tropical Medicine and International Health*, 9(11): 1228–38.

Bates, M.S. (1978) Ethnicity and pain: a bio-cultural model. *Social Science & Medicine*, 24: 47–50.

Berry, J.W. (1998) Acculturation and health. In: S.S. Kazarian and D.R. Evans (eds), *Cultural Clinical Psychology*. Oxford: Oxford University Press.

British Heart Foundation (2005) *2005 Coronary Heart Disease Statistics*. London: British Heart Foundation.

Broom, A. (2004) Prostate cancer and masculinity in Australian society: a case of stolen identity? *International Journal of Men's Health*, 3: 73–92.

Callister, L.C. (2003) Cultural influences on pain perceptions and behaviours. *Home Health Care Management and Practice*, 15(3): 207–11.

Chapple, A. & Ziebland, S. (2002) Prostate cancer: embodied experience and perceptions of masculinity. *Sociology of Health & Illness*, 24(6): 820 41.

Connell, R. (2000) *The Men and the Boys*. St Leonards, NSW: Allen & Unwin.

Connell, R.W. (2005) *Masculinities* (2nd edn). Cambridge: Polity.

Connell, R.W. & Messerschmidt, J.W. (2005) Hegemonic masculinity: rethinking the concept. *Gender and Society*, 19(6): 829–59.

Courtenay, W.H. (2000) Constructions of masculinity and their influence on men's well-being: a theory of gender and health, *Social Science & Medicine*, 50(10): 1385–401.

Emslie, C. (2005) Women, men and coronary heart disease: a review of the qualitative literature. *Journal of Advanced Nursing*, 51(4): 382–95.

Emslie, C., Ridge, D., Ziebland, S. and Hunt, K. (2006) Men's accounts of depression: reconstructing or resisting hegemonic masculinity? *Social Science & Medicine*, 62: 2246–57.

Evans, J., Butler, L., Etowa, J., Crawley, I., Rayson, D. & Bell, D.G. (2005) Gendered and cultured relations: exploring African Nova Scotians' perceptions and experiences of breast and prostate cancer. *Research and Theory for Nursing Practice: An International Journal*, 19(3): 257–73.

Franklin, C.W. (1984) *The Changing Definition of Masculinity*. New York: Plenum Press.

Galdas, P.M., Cheater, F.M. & Marshall, P. (2005) Men and health help-seeking behaviour: literature review. *Journal of Advanced Nursing*, 319(7207): 616–23.

Galdas, P.M., Cheater, F.M. & Marshall, P. (2007) What is the role of masculinity in white and South Asian men's decisions to seek medical help for cardiac chest pain? *Journal of Health Services Research Policy*, 12(4): 223–9.

Gascoigne, P. & Whitear, B. (1999) Making sense of testicular cancer symptoms: a qualitative study of the way in which men sought help from the health care services. *European Journal of Oncology Nursing*, 3(2): 62–9.

George, A. & Fleming, P. (2004) Factors affecting men's help-seeking in the early detection of prostate cancer: implications for health promotion. *Journal of Men's Health & Gender*, 1(4): 345–52.

GISSI (Gruppo Italiano per lo Studio Della Streptochiniasi Nell'Infarto Miocardico) (1986) Effectiveness of intravenous thrombolytic treatment in acute myocardial infarction. *Lancet*, 1: 397–401.

GISSI (Gruppo Italiano per lo Studio Della Streptochiniasi Nell'Infarto Miocardico)-Avoidable Delay Group (1995) Epidemiology of avoidable delay in the care of patients with acute myocardial infarction in Italy. *Archives of Internal Medicine*, 155(14): 1481–8.

Gough, B. (2006) 'Try to be healthy, but don't forgo your masculinity': deconstructing men's health discourse in the media, *Social Science & Medicine*, 63: 2476–88.

Gray, R.E., Fitch, M., Phillips, C., Labrecque, M. & Fergus, K. (2000) To tell or not to tell: patterns of disclosure among men with prostate cancer. *Psycho-Oncology*, 9: 273–82.

Grover, A., Kumar, R. & Jindal, S.K. (2003) Treatment-seeking behaviour of chest symptomatics. *Indian Journal of Tuberculosis*, 150(1): 87–92.

Hearn, J. & Collinson, D.L. (1994) Theorizing unities and difference between men and between masculinities. In H. Brod and M. Kaufman (eds), *Theorizing Masculinities*. London: Sage.

ISIS-2 (1988) Second international study of infarct survival. Collaborative group randomised trial of intravenous streptokinase, oral aspirin, both, or neither in 17,187 cases of suspected acute myocardial infarction. *Lancet*, 2: 349–60.

Joshi, P., Islam, S., Pais, P., Reddy, S., Dorairaj, P., Kazmi, K., Pandey, M.R., Haque, S., Mendis, S., Rangarajan, S. & Yusuf, S. (2007) Risk factors for early myocardial infarction in South Asians compared with individuals in other countries. *Journal of the American Medical Association*, 297(3): 286–94.

Kimmel, M.S. (1996) *Manhood in America*. New York: Free Press.

Lavery, J.F. and Clark, V.A. (1999) Prostate cancer: patients' and spouses' coping and marital adjustment. *Psychology, Health & Medicine*, 4: 289–302.

Mac an Ghaill, M. (1994) The making of black English masculinities. In H. Brod and M. Kaufman (eds), *Theorizing Masculinities*. London: Sage

Majors, R. & Billson, J.M. (1992) *Cool Pose: The Dilemmas of Black Manhood in America*. New York: Touchstone.

Montes-Sadoval, L. (2000) An analysis of the concept of pain. *Journal of Advanced Nursing*, 29: 935–41.

Morankar, S. & Weiss, M.G. (2003) Impact of gender in illness experience and behaviour: implications for tuberculosis control in rural Maharashtra. *Health Administrator*, 45(1&2): 149–55.

Nair, S.S., Radhakrishna, S., Seetha, M.A. & Rupert Samuel, G.E. (2002) Behaviour patterns of persons with chest symptoms in Karnataka state. *Indian Journal of Tuberculosis*, 49(1): 39–48.

Nayak, S., Shiflett, S.C., Eshun, S. & Levine, F.M. (2000) Culture and gender effects in pain beliefs and the prediction of pain tolerance. *Cross-Cultural Research*, 34: 135–51.

Norris, R.M. (1998) Fatality outside hospital from acute coronary events in three British health districts. *British Medical Journal*, 316: 1065–70.

O'Brien, R., Hunt, K. & Hart, G. (2005) 'It's caveman stuff, but that is to a certain extent how guys still operate': men's accounts of masculinity and help-seeking. *Social Science & Medicine*, 61(3): 503–16.

Oliffe, J.L. (2005) Prostatectomy induced impotence and masculinity. *Social Science & Medicine*, 60: 2249–59.

Oliffe, J.L., Grewal, S., Bottorff, J.L., Luke, H. and Toor, H. (2007) Elderly South Asian Canadian immigrant men: confirming and disrupting dominant discourses about masculinity and men's health. *Family & Community Health*, 30(3): 224–36.

Radley, A. (1994) *Making Sense of Illness: The Social Psychology of Health and Disease*. London: Sage.

Rich J.A. & Stone, D.A. (1996) The experience of violent injury for young African-American men: the meaning of being a 'sucker'. *Journal of General Internal Medicine*, 11: 77–82.

Robertson, S. (2006) 'Not living life in too much of an excess': lay men understanding health and well-being. *Health*, 10(2): 175–89.

Shaikh, B.T. & Hatcher, J. (2005) Health-seeking behaviour and health service utilisation in Pakistan: challenging the policy makers. *Journal of Public Health*, 27(1): 49–54.

Sheth, T., Nair, C., Nargundkar, M., Anand, S. & Yusuf, S. (1999) Cardiovascular and cancer mortality among Canadians of European, South Asian and Chinese origin from 1979–1993: an analysis of 1.2 million deaths. *Canadian Medical Association Journal*, 161: 132–8.

UKHAS (United Kingdom Heart Study) Collaborative Group (1998) Effect of time from onset to coming under care on fatality of patients with acute myocardial infarction: effect of resuscitation and thrombolytic treatment. *Heart*, 80: 114–20.

Wall, D. & Kristjanson, L. (2005) Men, culture and hegemonic masculinity: understanding the experience of prostate cancer. *Nursing Inquiry*, 12(2): 87–97.

White, A.K. & Johnson, M. (2000) Men making sense of their chest pain – niggles, doubts and denials. *Journal of Clinical Nursing*, 9(4): 534–41.

Yusuf, S., Hawken, S., Ounpuu, S., Dans, T., Avezum, A., Lanas, F., McQueen, M., Budaj, A., Pais, P., Varigos, J. & Lisheng, L. (2004) Effect of potentially modifiable risk factors associated with myocardial infarction in 52 countries (the INTER-HEART study): case-control study. *Lancet*, 364(9438): 937–52.

Yusuf, S., Reddy, S., Ounpuu, S. & Anand, S. (2001) Global burden of cardiovascular diseases. Part II: Variations in cardiovascular disease by specific ethnic groups and geographic regions and prevention strategies. *Circulation*, 104: 2855–64.

Zborowski, M. (1952) Cultural components in responses to pain. *Journal of Social Issues*, 8:16–30.

AFTERWORD: WHAT NEXT FOR MEN'S HEALTH RESEARCH?

The impetus for this book came from our recognition that critical perspectives relating to men, masculinities and health have been developing for some time, though often within different disciplinary silos and from within different countries. This has led to a situation where information, and opportunities for learning, are often 'lost' between disciplines as they talk past, rather than to, each other (an issue highlighted well in Chapter 1). Our overarching purpose here, therefore, was to bring some of this work together and provide a varied collection of such critical insights on the complex relationships between men, masculinities and health. Consequently, we make no apologies for the fact that this book has an eclectic feel to it, with work coming from cultural studies, psychology, sociology, anthropology, social policy and nursing. Neither do we apologise if methodological or theoretical frameworks between some chapters contradict each other. The intention was never to provide a uniform voice but rather to provoke and promote further discussion and debate within this area of work. That said, it is important here to consider what some of the main emerging themes have been from across and within the three parts of the book and to look at what questions and directions these might suggest for future work.

The contradictory and shifting nature of men's health 'behaviours', 'performances' or 'practices' is a major theme throughout the book. From the opening chapter's discussion of managing the 'superhero/schlemiel dyad', through consideration of the way that older men negotiate a 'don't care/should care' approach to health practices (Chapter 6), to the way that men with prostate cancer (Chapter 10) and chest pain (Chapter 12) engage with health care services and treatment options, there is strong emphasis on the fluid nature of men's health practices. While mainstream health professional texts have begun to recognise the importance of diversity (rather than homogeneity) among men (for example Banks, 2001; White, 2008), this is still often presented in terms of how different 'groups' of men respond to health messages, interventions or illness, or how *some* men manage to break out of traditional stereotypes. What is apparent from the work within this book is that the situation is more complex. Health and illness practices do not simply vary across groups of men or between individual men. Rather, such practices can vary in the same man at different times and in different locations. In short, it seems clear from the work presented here that men's health practices are socially contingent, dependent (though not determined) by a range of factors that include the impact of 'health' and 'gender' discourses (Chapters 5 and 7), access to material and physical resources (Chapters 3 and 8) and the ability and desire to maintain an embodied self that meets normative standards (Chapter 11). These factors were recognised as being interwoven in many of the chapters here.

Part of the ability to recognise this fluidity in men's practices lies in the way that 'masculinity' or 'masculinities' are conceptualised in relation to health and illness, and this represents another key feature of the book. While biomedicine has (mainly) moved away from wholly genetic/hormonal explanations for 'the way men are' (for their 'masculinity'), there is still a tendency to see 'masculinity' as something (character type, personality traits) men 'possess' in greater or lesser measure. Yet, even when accepting that socialisation plays a role in the construction of male gender, this is often interpreted as the 'amount' of stereotypical male characteristics or personality attributes individual men have been socialised with. (Indeed, there are a whole range of 'masculinity scales' designed to quantify this information or to capture similar information about the 'amount' of dissonance men experience between such stereotypes and their own ability to meet them.) Relationships (correlations) are then drawn between the degree to which men possess, or subscribe to, traditional male characteristics and their health and illness practices. The commonest relationship drawn is that the more traditional masculinity a man has been socialised into (i.e. the greater amount he has) the more likely he is to engage in a range of negative (risk-taking) health practices and therefore to suffer the health outcome consequences. As others have highlighted (Macdonald, 2006), such an approach to understanding masculinity can

obscure other significant determinants of men's health practices and outcomes. The fluid nature of men's health and illness practices, highlighted above, stems from recognition in the
contributions here that masculinity is not a set of attributes or
characteristics possessed by men. While there is certainly not full
agreement across the chapters about exactly how 'masculinity'
is to be understood, what is clear is that it is seen as a dynamic
force (or forces) that act upon and through men; that is to say,
'masculinities' are recognised as both the producer and product of gendered structures and men's agency. While this view of
masculinities is far from new, its application to work in men and
health has remained limited and dispersed to date (Chapter 1).

It is not just the social construction of gender and masculinities that are seen as significant. The meanings and values that
are attached to 'health' and 'healthy lifestyle' (Chapter 3), and
the way that physical and mental states become constructed as
'pathological' (Chapters 7 and 9), are also key issues of importance within the book, illuminating the contested and political
nature of men's health. The issue of 'gatekeeping' in interviews
with men around their health (Chapter 4) further elucidates
the importance of power relations and how 'health' and 'illness'
meaning is constructed, and resisted, and for whose ends and
purpose.

These three key emerging themes – the contradictory (fluid)
nature of men's social (health) practices; the recognition of
'masculinities' as sets (patterns) of social practices rather than
personal characteristics; and the way that 'health' and 'healthy
lifestyle' discourses carry socially constructed and politically contested meaning – suggest particular priorities for future work.
For *research*, we need to know more about which particular social
contexts facilitate or inhibit men's engagement in specific health-
related practices, why, and for which men. In particular, more
work needs to be completed that explores how different configurations of masculinities act to initiate such facilitation or
inhibition *and* how particular configurations of masculinities are
(re)produced within health professional interventions and forms
of service delivery. To do this work also requires a research
emphasis on deconstructing the discourses that surround meanings attached to both 'health', and 'gender/masculinities', and
their intersection. In the *practice* of health work with men, there
needs to be more application of what we already know about the

social contexts which generate, sustain and facilitate positive health practices for men and how best to utilise these opportunities; that is, there needs to be knowledge transfer of current evidence into practice. To do so requires recognising and valuing the positive aspects of particular configurations of masculinities and the positive contributions that men do make to their own health (and that of others), as well as how best to ameliorate the more negative aspects. There are also implications here relating to *policy*. The fluid and socially contingent nature of men's health practices, and the need to see 'masculinities' as other than personal characteristics, challenge an individual 'behaviour change' model for addressing men's health. There needs to be a development of public health/health promotion policies that recognise the relationship of social determinants and inequalities to the configurations of masculinities that men engage in and their subsequent health practices and outcomes. The complexity of the interrelations of social class, ethnicity, sexuality, disability and so forth to masculinities and health practices currently remain insufficiently researched but also under-recognised in the development of policy and practice in health work with men.

There is clearly much to be done in expanding the work on critical perspectives on men, masculinities and health. This collection opens the debates and highlights some of the issues yet remains only a starting point. We have provided views here from a particular Euro-Australian-North American standpoint. As others have recently highlighted (Connell, 2007) we need to be increasingly willing to incorporate views from outwith this dominant axis. If we are to move forward in areas where there is currently an impasse (such as gender inequalities in health – Annandale & Hunt, 2000) then we need to recognise the important and vital contributions to world social science that 'Southern Theory' can make. Future work in critical perspectives on men, masculinities and health needs also to incorporate a focus on this potential contribution.

REFERENCES

Annandale, E. & Hunt, K. (2000) *Gender Inequalities in Health: Research at the Crossroads*. In Annandale & Hunt (eds), *Gender Inequalities in Health*. Buckingham: Open University Press.

Banks, I. (2001) No man's land: men, illness and the NHS. *British Medical Journal*, 323: 1058–60.

Connell, R. (2007) *Southern Theory: The Global Dynamics of Knowledge in Social Science.* Cambridge: Polity.

Macdonald, J. (2006) Shifting paradigms: a social-determinants approach to solving problems in men's health policy and practice. *Medical Journal of Australia*, 185(8): 456–8.

White, A.K. (2008) Men and the problem of help seeking. In J.J. Heidelbaugh, *Clinical Men's Health: Evidence in Practice.* Philadelphia: Saunders Elsevier.

INDEX